HOW TO STOP THE PAIN

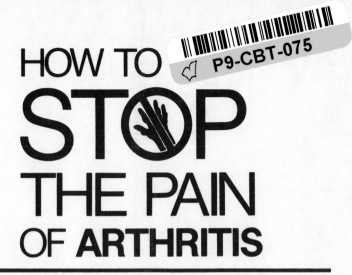

P9-CBT-075

OF ARTHRITIS

The discovery that the commercial medical establishment tried to suppress - without success!

The Authors
Professor Henry B. Rothblatt, J.D., L.L.M.
Donna Pinorsky, R.N., B.A.
Michael Brodsky, Editor, ARTHRITIS Nutrition Aging News
with The Medical Committee of the Institute for Research of
Rheumatic Diseases

Published by
COMPACT BOOKS, INC.
P.O. Box 6263
Hollywood, Florida 33021
Copyright© 1984 by COMPACT BOOKS

All rights reserved. No part of this book may be reproduced
in any form or by any means whatsoever without the prior
written permission of the Publisher, excepting brief quotes
used in connection with reviews written
specifically for inclusion in a magazine or newspaper.

Library of Congress #84-061541

TABLE OF CONTENTS

Chapter I

What Is Arthritis And How Can It Do Such Damage To The Human Body?

*A*ny meaningful discussion of the various forms of arthritis disease which affect millions of Americans must begin with those body structures essential to movement of the joints.

What is a joint and what does it do?

A few joints of the body furnish a permanent union of bones in the skeletal system and contribute to overall body stability. However, most joints unite bones in a less rigid manner to allow for body movement. These joints are called **synovial joints.**

1

Synovial joints have the following features:

1) a joint cavity or space located between the two ends of cartilage-covered bones which are flexibly united to form the joint.

2) an inner synovial membrane or lining that produces the lubricating joint fluid. An outer fibrous lining also combines with the inner synovial membrane to form the joint capsule. This tough fibrous capsule keeps the joint together.

3) the bone ends are covered by joint cartilage.

Movement in the joints takes place when one cartilage-covered bone end moves over the other. Bone never moves directly over bone. The tough but elastic cartilage cushions movement by serving as a kind of shock absorber in weight-bearing joints.

Joint cartilage has neither a nerve nor a blood supply. Cartilage is nourished by the small blood vessels in bone and by the synovial fluid.

Joints can move in many different directions and in many different ways. Most of our movements, however, are complicated combinations of simple movements.

RHEUMATOID ARTHRITIS

In rheumatoid arthritis, the linings of affected joints become inflamed — painful, swollen, red and hot. Actually, inflammation first affects the blood vessels that feed into the joint lining which thickens and swells. The joint lining then produces more lubricating fluid which can form a sticky fibrous layer between cartilage-covered bone ends. This formation is known as a **pannus.**

If the pannus persists, then the exposed cartilage will gradually be destroyed both by the pannus and the inflamed blood vessels. Cells in the joint lining will die and liberate enzymes, proteins that affect the rate of chemical reactions without being altered themselves in the process, that eat away at protein-dependent tissue.

As cartilage is broken down, the joint becomes unfit for normal use. The joint can be forced to move in unintended directions it was not structured for. This forced movement increases injury and pain and leads to crippling deformity and disfigurement. Bone ends may fuse to produce a stiff joint.

SIGNS AND SYMPTOMS OF RHEUMATOID ARTHRITIS

It has been estimated that approximately 5 million Americans suffer from rheumatoid arthritis.

Rheumatoid arthritis predominantly affects the joints, but other organs, such as the heart, lungs, and nerves, may also become involved. The disease occurs two to three times more frequently in women than in men. All ages may be affected but the peak period of onset occurs between the ages of 25 and 35.

As pointed out by Fred G. Kantrowitz, M.D., Assistant Professor of Medicine at Harvard Medical School and Chief of the Rheumatology Unit at Beth Israel Hospital (MEDICAL TIMES, February 1982: "Grand Rounds from Beth Israel Hospital"), symptoms may begin five to ten years before the definitive onset of the disease!

The first early symptoms may be inflammation of a single joint. In some patients, injury, surgery, inoculation, infection or pregnancy may precede the first attack of rheumatoid arthritis.

The definitive onset usually takes the form of inflammation in several joints with few or no other symptoms. Most patients complain of morning stiffness diminishing through the course of the day. Frequently, stiffness comes back in the late afternoon or early evening. Patients may also suffer from an aching in the joints which interferes with sleep.

Virtually any joint, large or small, may be involved and this involvement is usually symmetrical. This means that if the right knee is affected then the left knee will probably also be involved. Two joints whose involvement in rheumatoid arthritis has not been thoroughly documented are the temporomandibular joint of the jaw, which often causes facial pain, and the cricoarytenoid joint of the throat. Involvement of this joint in rheumatoid arthritis produces hoarseness.

The ankles, elbows, shoulders and hips are often involved in rheumatoid arthritis.

Rheumatoid nodules occur in about 20% of all adult patients. They usually appear beneath the skin over pressure

3

points. These nodules are firm, non-tender, and probably result from inflammation of local blood vessels.

The hands are almost always affected by rheumatoid arthritis. There is frequently tenderness and swelling of the joints at the base of the fingers and of the set of finger joints nearest to these in early stages of the disease. The finger joints furtherest from the base of the fingers are almost never involved. In contrast, the small bones of the wrist are most often affected.

OSTEOARTHRITIS

Osteoarthritis is the most prevalent form of arthritis disease. Unlike rheumatoid arthritis, which occurs three times more frequently in women than in men, osteoarthritis occurs with equal frequency in both sexes.

This condition is closely related to the aging and cumulative wear-and-tear on joints. The exact sequence of events is still poorly understood. However, changes beneath the surface of joint cartilage seem to lead to flaking and cracks in the surface.

Several theories have been suggested to explain the changes in cartilage. Failure of lubrication, slow cumulative erosion of the surface cartilage, and fatigue of gradually stiffening cartilage due to inpact shock, are all possible causes.

Sometimes joints break down early because of biochemical changes in the body, there may be joints whose bone-ends are ill-fitting from birth. Congenital dislocation of the hip belongs in this category. Therefore, aging may not be the only cause of osteoarthritis.

After the surface cartilage begins to flake, deep clefts appear before the destruction of cartilage by enzymes lodged in the joint lining. W. Carson Dick, M.D. and W. Watson Buchann ("Osteoarthritis", REPORTS ON RHEUMATIC DISEASES, 1959-1977) are careful to point out that these changes must be carefully distinguished from those of simple aging. In simple aging, the water content of cartilage is lowered. In osteoarthritis, the water content stays the same or increases only negligibly.

These destructive changes in cartilage usually put a corresponding strain on bone in those areas where it is attached to muscle. The body responds to the strain by depositing extra calcium in the outer margin of bone and joint. These calcium deposits, called bony spurs (osteophytes), may accumulate over many years. When they affect the end row of finger joints they are known as Heberden's nodes, in honor of the British physician who first identified them in the eighteenth century.

With time, the combination of cartilage breakdown and spur formation can hamper normal joint functioning.

SIGNS AND SYMPTOMS OF OSTEOARTHRITIS

A person with advanced osteoarthritis may not necessarily suffer from pain because cartilage is not provided with nerves. The development of osteoarthritis is usually slow, with the body accommodating itself to erosion of cartilage and bony spurs over many years.

However, people with osteoarthritis can complain of pain and loss of joint function. Sudden and severe pain often occurs at night or after movement and minor injury. The lower spine, hips and knees are often the most painful osteoarthritic joints. In these joints, there is often great presure on neighboring tissues, muscles and ligaments.

When it affects the hand, osteoarthritis tends to appear most frequently in the end finger joints and in the joint at the base of the thumb.

Osteoarthritis of the knee occurs in about 30% of all cases of the disease, E.C. Huskisson and F.D. Hart, M.D. of Westminster Hospital, London, England (JOINT DISEASE: ALL THE ARTHROPATHIES, Year Book Medical Publishers, Inc.) This may account for the creaking noises (crepitus) audible with movement and the knees may become knobby and straighten out only with difficulty. Osteoarthritis secondary to overweight is often associated with the knees, as well as the big toes.

Unlike rheumatoid arthritis, osteoarthritis singles out and may cause tremendous pain and crippling to the hip joint. The hip joint allows for movement in all directions. When this joint is worn down by the osteoarthritis disease process, it is only able to bend backwards and forwards.

FOCUS ON ANKYLOSING SPONDYLITIS

The vertebral column, consists of 33 individual bones, maintains and supports the body in an erect position, pivots and allows for movement of the head, and gives the arms and legs a base from which to move.

The joints of the vertebral column, where the bones must also be joints, help keep it both rigid and flexible. Flexibility is necessary if the trunk is to move and proper balance and posture are to be maintained.

In ankylosing spondylitis, which occurs ten times more frequently in men than in women (M.I.V. Jayson and A.St.J. Dixon, Understanding Arthritis and Rheumatism, Dell Publishing Company, Inc.). The main symptom is inflammation of those sites where joint capsules and ligaments are attached to bones, especially in the spine.

Inflammation usually begins in the sacroiliac joints, which attach the sacrum (or tail bone) at the base of the spine to a bone of the pelvis. From the sacroiliac joints, inflammation may gradually spread up the spine to the neck region.

Inflammatory injury at these sites leads to destruction of ligaments and erosion of underlying bone. The body reacts by laying down bony spurs on the eroded bone, to which the ligaments reattach themselves. Ultimately, adjacent bones of the spine may connect rendering the joint stiff (ankylosed) and unfit for movement.

In many cases, ankylosing spondylitis is a disease of young men under thirty years of age. According to James Sharp, M.D. (ANKYLOSING SPONDYLITIS, Reports on Rheumatic Diseases, 1959-1977), about 60% of those afflicted complain of pain and stiffness in the lower back region. These discomforts may extend to the buttocks and back of the thigh.

In the early stages, severe stiffness and aching in the back may occur only in the early morning hours. If a truly effective therapy, i.e. the Holistic Balanced Treatment, is not introduced early enough, the spine will be bent forward permanently. Motion may become so limited that the patient finds it difficult to turn around or bend sideways or forward. Putting on socks and tying shoelaces become impossible tasks.

About 25% of those suffering from ankylosing spondylitis have arthritis in joints outside the spine. These tend to be the large joints of the shoulder, hips and knees, rather than the small joints of the fingers and feet. In juveniles, ankylosing spondylitis may present as arthritis of the hip or knee joints.

Iritis, inflammation of the iris of the eye, occurs in between one-fourth and one-third of people with ankylosing spondylitis. This condition, which is painful and causes blurring of vision, must be treated quickly and properly to avoid permanent injury. The Holistic Balanced Treatment has had great success in treating iritis.

Studies indicate that people who inherit specific HLA antigens have an enhanced susceptibility to certain diseases. Among these diseases are ragweed hay fever, psoriasis, multiple sclerosis and myasthenia gravis, as well an ankylosing spondylitis.

GOUTY ARTHRITIS

Gouty arthritis is characterized by the presence of tiny crystals in the joint fluid.

Chapter II
Causes
of Arthritis

*T*he cause or causes of arthritis are still not completely understood given the present state of our medical knowledge. Several factors—immunological, genetic, nutritional, bacterial— may interact to produce the various forms of the disease.

AN IMMUNOLOGICAL SLANT

There is considerable evidence to suggest that immunological reactions are very important in causing arthritis. An immunological reaction is one in which the body responds to invasion by such foreign organisms as viruses and bacteria through the production of protector proteins known as antibodies. When antibodies are doing their job properly, these foreign invaders are either inactivated or destroyed.

A large body of scientific evidence indicates that in rheumatoid arthritis the body's immune system may stop functioning properly. Instead the antibodies and other defense substances react against the body's own tissues as if they were foreign. Such reactions are classified as **autoimmune phenomena.**

Arthritis autoimmune phenomena may result in painful inflammation of the joints, lungs, skin, heart, blood and kidneys.

8

GENETICS AND THE DEVELOPMENT
OF RHEUMATOID ARTHRITIS

According to Dr. Nathan J. Zvaifler, speaking at an arthritis epidemiology conference held by the National Institute of Arthritis, Metabolism and Digestive Diseases (MEDICAL TRIBUNE), the presence of a substance called rheumatoid factor, found in the blood of many people with rheumatoid arthritis, is far more likely to indicate rheumatoid arthritis when it is found along with HLA-DR4 antigen. HLA-DR4 antigen is one of over 50 inherited substances identified on the surfaces of cells throughout the body.

It has been discovered that people who inherit specific HLA antigens are more likely to develop diseases such as psoriasis, multiple sclerosis, ragweed hayfever, and insulin-dependent diabetes, as well as many rheumatic diseases.

According to Derrick Brewerton, M.D. (REPORTS ON THE RHEUMATIC DISEASES), it is still unclear whether the HLA antigens are directly involved in the arthritis disease process or whether disease susceptibility results from the inheritance of weakened immunological defense associated with these specific HLA antigens.

IMPORTANT NEW LEADS THROUGH
RESEARCH STUDIES

In a study cited by Dr. Zvaifler, 52% of rheumatoid arthritis patients with rheumatoid factor also possessed the HLA-DR4 antigen. In contrast, only 25% of rheumatoid arthritis patients without rheumatoid factor possessed the HLA-DR4 antigen.

In the view of Dr. Elizabeth Barrett-Connor of the University of California School of Medicine at San Diego, the HLA-DR4 antigen is, at present, the "hottest" lead in the quest for genetic factor links to rheumatoid arthritis.

A VIRAL APPROACH TO THE DISEASE

In the view of Dr. Michael A. Catalano of the Scripps Clinic and Rehabilitation Foundation in La Jolla, California, the agent responsible for triggering the onset of rheumatoid arthritis (once a hereditary or genetic susceptibility is already present) may be a well-known virus. This organism, called the Epstein-Barr virus, is responsible for causing mononucleosis, an illness characterized by fever, sore throat, and lymph node and spleen distension.

The possibility of a connection between rheumatoid arthritis and viral or bacterial infection is not new. The inflammation, fever, increased heartbeat and abnormally large number of white blood cells present in the disease all suggest infection. However, until an infectious agent has been isolated in the blood of all arthritis sufferers, the assertion of an infectious cause of arthritis cannot be made definitively.

NUTRITION AND ARTHRITIS

The relation between diet and arthritis is indisputable. Many patients become aware of marked flare-ups in their arthritis symptoms after consumption of certain foods. Empty-caloried processed foods, refined sugar and refined sugar products, foods cured or spiced with salt, coffee, tea, caffeinated soft drinks, and tobacco are all capable of exacerbating arthritis symptoms.

In other words, the importance of diet in the management of arthritis cannot be overemphasized. A sound diet is crucial to the healing of arthritis-injured tissue and to optimum lifelong well-being.

However, this does not mean that nutritional factors or diet cause arthritis.

We might note that research in the area of the relation between food allergy and arthritis pain is increasing rapidly.

Dr. Marshall Mandell, medical director of the Alan Mandell Center for Bio-Ecologic Diseases, is one of a select group of health practitioners adventurous enough to chart the correlation between allergic symptoms, such as arthritis joint and muscle pain, depression, headache, fatigue, and bowel and bladder reactions, with the ingestion of certain foods. e.g. soybean, sugar, milk, coffee, egg, beef, ethanol, yeast, tobacco smoke.

ARTHRITIS: A DISEASE OF THE EMOTIONS

Another possibility is that arthritis is a disease of the emotions, a stress which ultimately affects the joints of the body. This is not unlikely given the interdependence of mind, body and emotions consistently considered in holistic approaches to well-being.

Researchers have recorded cases of rheumatoid arthritis triggered by intense emotional shock or trauma. It has also been shown that the course of the disease can be greatly influenced by worry, anxiety and fatigue. Family problems, loss of a loved one, and financial problems have been closely correlated with flare-ups of arthritis.

J.L. Halliday, a British researcher (LANCET) believes that arthritis is indeed a psychosomatic disorder in which emotional conflicts are expressed through somatic, or bodily, symptoms and sees the arthritis sufferer as a special personality type. Sometimes the person with arthritis tends to keep painful emotions bottled up, or repressed, inside, and tries to hide his or her problems from both himself or herself and others. When such a person is faced with additional stress or a life crisis, for example, physical danger or family tensions he or she may develop arthritis as the body's capacity for self-defense becomes exhausted and fails.

Halliday's theory is perhaps too extreme. Physicians skilled in administering the Holistic Balanced Treatment have become familiar with a broad spectrum of personality types over many years. However, strong emotion must certainly be considered an important component of the arthritis puzzle.

DR. HANS SELYE AND THE CONCEPT OF DISEASES OF ADAPTATION

Several decades ago, the concept of "diseases of adaption" was studied by Dr. Hans Selye, Director of the Institute of Experimental Medicine and Surgery at the University of Montreal in Canada.

Dr. Selye's revolutionary concept of disease focused less on germs and external agents and concentrated on a flawed internal response to stress.

In his writings and experimental work, the Canadian researcher always paid particular attention to arthritis as a disease of adaptation.

According to Selye, whatever primary disease producer is responsible for arthritis it is not very injurious in itself. Rather, it is the body's defective adaptation to the stressor in question which sets the debilitating symptomatology, inflammation, disfigurement, crippling, in motion.

CAUSATIVE FACTORS IN OSTEOARTHRITIS

Osteoarthritis, the most common form of arthritis, is so prevalent in the elderly that it has long been felt to be a typical manifestation of the aging process.

According to R.M. Acheson and A.B. Collart ("New Haven Survey of Joint Diseases XVII. Relationship Between Some Systemic Characteristics and Osteoarthritis in a General Population," ANNALS OF THE RHEUMATIC DISEASES, 1975), the way in which aging affects the onset of osteoarthritis is still not well understood.

PHYSICAL FACTORS AND OSTEOARTHRITIS

Several kinds of injury may affect joint cartilage.

One impact can cause an injury to joint cartilage. The injury may be followed by osteoarthritis, according to Jacques G. Peyron, M.D. ("Epidemiologic and Etiologic Approach to Osteoarthritis," SEMINARS IN ARTHRITIS AND RHEUMATISM, May, 1979). The role of single impact injury in the genesis of osteoarthritis has been demonstrated for the hip, knee, elbow and wrist joints.

Overactivity can also be a causative factor in osteoarthritis. For example, osteoarthritis of the hip has a 52% frequency among retired athletes, according to Y. Desmarais ("Hanche du Sportif", Paris). Hip osteoarthritis is also more prevalent in farming populations.

OBESITY AND OSTEOARTHRITIS

The work of Acheson and his colleagues has demonstrated that osteoarthritis is more prevalent in overweight people than in thin ones. Obesity by itself, however, does not appear to be an important factor in the onset and development of the majority of cases of osteoarthritis.

A recent study by R.H. Goldin and colleagues (ANNALS OF THE RHEUMATIC DISEASES) of osteoarthritis sufferers between the ages of 26 and 54 revealed that serious long-term excessive weight could not be correlated with early osteoarthritis in the knee, wrist, finger, hip, ankle and foot joints.

SPECIFIC CAUSATIVE FACTORS
ACCORDING TO SPECIFIC DISEASE SITE

There are two categories of finger osteoarthritis. In the first category, the distal interphalangeal joints (end finger joints) are generally involved. The principal causative factors are heredity and trauma. Heredity seems to play more of a role in women; trauma appears to be more decisive among men.

The other form of finger osteoarthritis is characterized by flare-ups in the joints furthest from the fingertips. The flare-ups are generally followed by remission and relapse. This leads to the wearing away of bone and, upon occasion, to serious destruction of the joints involved.

CAUSES OF OSTEOARTHRITIS IN THE KNEE

In knee osteoarthritis, as in hip osteoarthritis, a major role seems to be played by structural defects. Joint instability, resulting from ligament injury, and joint hypermobility are also considered significant causative agents in the development of knee osteoarthritis.

OSTEOARTHRITIS OF THE SHOULDER

Osteoarthritis rarely occurs in the shoulder region and is usually observed after age 60. Serious injury of joint tissue is considered a major cause. Excessive use of the shoulder joint may also be a factor of importance, for example, shoulder osteoarthritis is frequently seen among professional hunters.

It is important to point out that, at present, the list of causative factors in osteoarthritis is still very incomplete. We do not know the mechanisms employed by these factors to effect the breakdown of joint cartilage, nor do we know how these factors interact. It is very possible that heredity and occupation combine with certain biochemical factors to produce the clinical picture in osteoarthritis.

ARE CRYSTALS THE CULPRIT

British researchers from the Department of Experimental Pathology, Medical College of London, England, (MEDICAL TRIBUNE) believe that a mineral crystal deposited in certain joints may be the real culprit in osteoarthritis.

According to Dr. Willoughby, Director of Research and Rheumatology, an inherited metabolic disorder, responsible for the breakdown of the body's calcium balance, leads to calcium crystal deposition in various joints. The calcium deposits cause inflammation and injury to joint cartilage.

Although it is unlikely that these calcium deposits are the primary causative factor in osteoarthritis, the research carried out by the British scientists is significant for the role it suggests in the interaction of heredity and biochemical metabolism.

Chapter III

A Straightforward Look At The Other Drugs For Arthritis

A drug may be defined as any substance, other than a food, used in the prevention, healing, treatment or cure of disease in man or in animals.

Side effects are produced when a drug prescribed for a particular purpose affects the body in ways that are totally unconnected with that purpose.

As pointed out by Louis S. Goodman, M.D., Sc.D., and Alfred Gilman, Ph.D. (THE PHARMACOLOGICAL BASIS OF THERAPEUTICS, The Macmillan Company, 970), no drug is free of toxic, or harmful, side effects. These effects may be insignificant, but they sometimes turn out to be quite serious and even fatal.

Arthritis drugs are therapeutic agents whose target is the various arthritis diseases, rheumatoid arthritis, osteoarthritis, ankylosing spondylitis, gouty arthritis, juvenile rheumatoid arthritis and psoriatic arthritis. All the conventional arthritis drugs produce side effects. Very frequently, these side effects prove to be highly damaging, even devastating. In contrast, the Holistic Balanced Treatment works in harmony with the body: when side effects do occur with this dynamic threefold approach they are not life-threatening.

All patients, not only arthritis sufferers, must be made aware of the reality of drug-induced illness, especially today, with the number of drugs growing at an alarming rate and drug companies channelling greater and greater sums into publicity for new products in the hope of vast profits.

As David H. McCallum, a health industry analyst at the prestigious investment firm of Paine, Webber, Mitchell & Hutchins, has pointed out ("The Boom in Arthritis Drugs", THE NEW YORK TIMES, Friday, April 23, 1982), no conventional arthritis drug really works very well. This state of affairs triggers a "high level of switching from one drug to another". Such frenzied shuttling from drug to drug on the part of desperate arthritis sufferers is what makes the arthritis drug industry a $700 million a year market.

Why do side effects occur? Why can a drug like penicillin produce, in the course of its battle against infection, such symptoms as vomiting, nausea, diarrhea, skin eruptions, itchings,, and, in some cases, sudden death? Why does Valium, employed against anxiety, lead to drowsiness, constipation, skin rashes, insomnia, and even cancer?

Many or most drugs are non-specific. They do not focus on one target organ or tissue within the body. For example, drug X may succeed in eradicating a specific bacterial infection, and at the same time, destroy another strain of bacteria located in the intestine which helps synthesize essential vitamins.

The elderly are especially sensitive to the side effects of drugs. Any drug is effective for a limited time only and, under normal circumstances, by the time its effectiveness is over it has been broken down (metabolized) and excreted through stool or urine. Due to wear and tear on the system, older people may not be able to break drugs down for excretion in an efficient manner. Even normal therapeutic dosages may pose a problem. As a result, an unwanted accumulation of these chemicals in the body may result, leading to illness.

Unlike the other drugs for arthritis, the Holistic Balanced Treatment has a specific focus and a specific effect. This innovative combination of prednisone, testosterone and estradiol does not merely mask symptoms as the arthritis disease progresses unchecked to cause painful crippling, disfigurement and deformity, and, often irrevocable injury to skin, heart, lungs and nerves. The Holistic Balanced Treatment confronts the underlying arthritis disease in a straightforward manner so that the body can go on to heal itself and achieve optimum lifelong health.

Before we examine the grave side effects of the various arthritis drugs, it is useful to list the basic categories of drug-related injury:

A) Drug allergy. Drug allergy can take various forms, including skin reactions, asthma, inflammation of the nasal mucous membrane (rhinitis), and injury to liver cells.

B) Blood dyscrasias, or appearance of abnormal material in the blood. The white blood cell count might be strikingly lower than normal, and, in some cases, there are significant defects in the bloodclotting factors.

C) Liver and kidney injury.

D) Injurious effects on behavior. These may include reduction in motivation, memory and learning impairment, inappropriate behavior, and disturbances in motor coordination.

E) Drug dependence or addiction.

F) Drug poisoning.

ASPIRIN

The harmful side effects of aspirin are not as well known as they should be.

Aspirin is able to lessen the pain and inflammation of rheumatoid arthritis for only brief periods of time before incre ed doses are needed.

Aspirin is known to cause STOMACH AND INTESTINAL BLEEDING, ANEMIA, a life-threatening allergic reaction known as ANAPHYLACTIC SHOCK, SWELLING, HIVES and ASTHMA.

Mere therapeutic doses of aspirin can produce DEAFNESS and VERTIGO (dizziness). Small single doses have been

17

associated with SHOCK, BRONCHIOLAR CONSTRICTION, narrowing of the very fine subdivisions of the bronchial tubes of the pulmonary system, and RHINORRHEA, a watery discharge from the nose.

If the amount of aspirin administered is greater than 1 gram/lb. one may expect harmful stimulation of the central nervous system, followed by DEPRESSION and CONFUSION. CONVULSIONS have, in some cases, been succeeded by COMA and STUPOR, HALLUCINATIONS and PARANOIA.

According to two University of Pennsylvania researchers, Dr. Martin Goldberg and Dr. Thomas Murray, mixing aspirin and another pain reliever, phenacetin, has a markedly unhealthy effect on the kidney and is a possible cause of chronic kidney disease. Mixing the two painkillers account for 5% of all deaths from kidney failure each year.

Several cases of babies born "blue" with pulmonary hypertension and hypoxia (decreased oxygen) have been traced to aspirin intake by their mothers during pregnancy. These cases were reported by Drs. Abraham H. Rudolph of the University of California at San Francisco and Daniel L. Levin of the University of Texas at Dallas (MEDICAL WORLD NEWS).

Medical professionals who testified at a Senate hearing in 1978 urged consumers to be on guard against the stomach problems aspirin is all too capable of creating, especially the possibility of STOMACH ULCERS.

According to Dr. Elliott Sagall, Medical Education Director for the American Trial Lawyers Association, aspirin may be capable of inducing "fresh ulcerations."

The person with arthritis must take aspirin throughout the day, day in and day out to attain some relief. As a result of regular intake, aspirin levels build up—dangerously—in the blood. Drs. Sahud and Cohen of the University of California Department of Medicine have pointed out in the respected British medical journal LANCET how these high blood levels of aspirin can affect the body. For one thing, they lead to a significant depletion of vitamin C in platelets and plasma (the clear, acellular portion of the blood).

The person with arthritis must take aspirin throughout the day, day in and day out to attain some relief. As a result of

18

regular intake, aspirin levels build up—dangerously—in the blood. Drs. Sahud and Cohen of the University of California Department of Medicine have pointed out in the respected British medical journal LANCET how these high blood levels of aspirin can affect the body. For one thing they lead to a significant depletion of vitamin C in platelets and plasma, the clear, acellular portion of the blood.

Blood platelets keep us from losing large, and in some cases fatal, quantities of blood after injury. When a wound breaks through the wall of a blood vessel, platelets come to the rescue by sticking (adhering) to each other and thereby covering up, through aggregation, the health-threatening breach.

Aspirin interferes with the ability of platelets to adhere to each other. By binding to individual platelets, aspirin prevents their essential binding to each other.

Aspirin can have an adverse effect on platelet adhesion or clumping for as long as 8 days. According to Dr. Theodore Spaet of the Albert Einstein College of Medicine in New York City, one dose of aspirin can destroy platelet-clumping capacity. Eventually, these damaged platelets are replaced by new healthy ones. However, if aspirin intake continues unabated at the rate of tablets twice daily, overall platelet functioning will remain ineffective despite the constant turnover.

Dr. James Roth of the University of Pennsylvania has demonstrated that aspirin makes 60% of all users bleed internally. In some cases, large quantities of blood are lost.

The lowering of vital vitamin C levels in especially dangerous for the person with rheumatoid arthritis since capillary fragility (easy bruising) is a conspicuous tendency in this condition. When aspirin intake provokes vitamin C depletion, the ability of this vitamin to prevent and repair capillary fragility as well as petechiae, pinpoint hemorrhages on the surface of the skin, in consequently lost.

Vitamin C is also essential in maintaining the structural integrity of cartilage and bone. Without adequate vitamin C levels, we are exposed to an enhanced risk of fracture.

IBUPROFEN OR MOTRIN

Motrin belongs to the class of nonsteroidal anti-inflammatory agents (NSAIDS). Incapable of affecting the underlying course of arthritis disease, Mortin only relieves pain, ignoring the continuing deterioration and wasting of tissue.

Like aspirin, ibuprofen, or Motrin as it is known commercially, is derived from a class of substances known as organic acids.

Though less effective as an anti-inflammatory agent than aspirin, Motrin has been presented as an effective alternative to the marked gastrointestinal bleeding linked to aspirin intake. Unfortunately, as the dosage of this agent is increased to elicit the desired, but all too fleeting anti-inflammatory effect, Motrin begins to reveal undesirable side effects.

These include PEPTIC ULCERATION, BLURRED and REDUCED VISION, RETINAL DAMAGE, and, ironically enough, GASTROINTESTINAL BLEEDING!

Studies indicate that the most common side effect of Motrin use is GASTROINTESTINAL UPSET, NAUSEA, VOMITING, and PAIN in the pit of the stomach. In one study, gastrointestinal problems appeared in 4-16% of all Motrin users.

DIZZINESS, NERVOUSNESS, HEADACHE, SKIN RASH, DECREASED APPETITE, and TINNITUS (ringing in the ears) have also been reported. A cause-and-effect relation between Motrin and DEPRESSION and INSOMNIA as well as URTICARIA, hives, has been suggested on several occasions. There is even a possibility that Motrin may be linked to HEPATITIS and other instances of abnormal liver functioning, HALLUCINATIONS, ALOPECIA (hair loss), CONJUNCTIVITIS, BLEEDING EPISODES, LUPUS ERYTHEMATOSUS, ARRHYTHMIAS (defective heart rhythms), and HYPOGLYCEMIA.

The Upjohn Company, manufacturer of Motrin, has pointed out that several serious blood disturbances may stem from Motrin consumption. These include decrease in the white blood cell count, decrease in hemoglobin (anemia, low blood), and increase in bleeding time.

BUTAZOLIDIN ALKA OR PHENYLBUTAZONE

Butazolidin is longer-acting than aspirin but is also more toxic.

According to Meyers, Jawetz and Goldfien, authors of the REVIEW OF MEDICAL PHARMACOLOGY, "the contraindications and cautions made a part of the labelling by the manufacturer are so stringent and comprehensive than responsibility for any adverse result of therapy would probably devolve on the physician."

These adverse effects and contraindications are all too typical of painkillers like butazolidin. First, butazolidin is not recommended for rheumatoid arthritis patients who have EDEMA, CARDIAC PROBLEMS, BLOOD DYSCRASIAS, or DRUG ALLERGY. In addition, butazolidin must be used with great caution when the patient exhibits HIGH BLOOD PRESSURE, LIVER DAMAGE, PEPTIC ULCER, and URINARY INCOMPETENCE. At higher doses the side effects of the drug include SODIUM AND FLUID RETENTION, DRY MOUTH, VOMITING, NAUSEA, PEPTIC ULCER, HEMORRHAGE and LIVER DAMAGE, as well as SKIN INFLAMMATION.

According to Ciga-Geigy, cases of leukemia have been observed in patients using this drug over both the short and the long-term. Most of the victims were over 40 years of age.

About 5% of all patients treated with butazolidin develop a skin lesion consisting of macropapules (pimples). When a RASH occurs, the drug should be promptly discontinued.

There is one case in the medical literature of a 53-year old man who was advised to take butzolidin for his arthritis. He developed Stevens-Johnson syndrome, producing permanent blindness, after taking the drug for only 2 weeks. He subsequently received only a $500,000 settlement from the butzolidin drug manufacturer and the physician who prescribed the drug.

In another case, a college football player developed bone marrow damage, chronic anemia, and chronic mononucleosis after taking butazolidin prescribed by the team physician. Within four years of graduation, these illnesses had worsened to a point where he was forced to go on disability. There are many other cases of patients who have died as a result of the peptic ulcerations, cardiovascular complications, liver damage and leukemia triggered by butazolidin use.

THE CASE AGAINST INDOCIN (INDOMETHACIN)

Like butazolidin, Indocin is not suggested for general use as a pain reliever. It is used only in special situations. It causes fewer serious side effects than butazolidin but the range of undesirable reactions is wider.

First, Indocin is contraindicated for children under 14 years of age, pregnant and nursing mothers, victims of gastrointestinal tract injury, and people with allergic reactions to aspirin. Indocin users often expereince HIGHLY SEVERE GASTROINTESTINAL REACTIONS to the drug. According to a printout issued to physicians by the manufacturers of Indocin "the prescribing physician must be continuously alert for any sign or symptom signalling a possible gastrointestinal reaction" due to the "severity of gastrointestinal reactions to Indocin."

As reported in **The People's Doctor,** A Medical Newsletter for Consumers (Volume 2, Number 3), written by Robert S. Mendelsohn M.D., Indocin may also produce symptoms of COMA, LOSS OF BALANCE, SUSCEPTIBILITY to HALLUCINATIONS, and GRADUAL BLINDNESS

Other side effects include HEADACHES, DEPRESSION, CONFUSION, DIZZINESS, and SLEEPINESS, as well as HAIR LOSS.

Because of its high potency, Indocin poses a very real threat to the integrity of the central nervous system. PSYCHIATRIC PROBLEMS, CONVULSIONS and PARKINSONISM have occurred with administration of this drug. Due to the adverse effect on nervous system functioning, patients receiving Indocin are counselled not to drive or perform activities requiring alertness or concentrated effort.

Another, and by no means insignificant, danger of Incodin use is its capacity to hide typical signs of infection. During Indocin administration, the prescribing physician must be especially alert to signs of infection camouflaged by the drug.

Death as a result of hemorrhage and ulceration of stomach and small intestine has been noted with Indocin. This drug has also been linked with ULCERATIVE COLITIS, HEPATITIS, JAUNDICE and ASTHMA.

Merck and Company, one of the largest drug companies, has called a temporary halt to foreign sales of the sustained-release version of Indocin. This version of the drug supposedly releases small quantities over a given time period.

Merck's suspension of Indocin (indomethacin) sales, which occurred in early September (MARKET PLACE, POSITIVE VIEWS ABOUT MERCK, NY TIMES, September 14, 1983) took place in response to reports of unexpected side effects.

News of the dangerous side effects of the drug caused a 4⅝ point drop in Merck stock on September 1, 1983. However, David M. Paisley, drug analyst for Merill Lynch, counselled the firm's clients to view the drop as an opportunity to buy! Another presitgious investment firm, Smith Barney, Harris, Upham and Company reacted similarly to Merck's indomethacin-related "weakness', uring investors to lose no time in buying the company's stock at an attractive lower price. Smith Barney has also added Merck to the "growth category of its recommended list" as a result of the drop.

David K. Crossen, drug analyst for Smith Barney, estimates Merck earnings at $6.14 per share during this year and predicts a figure of $7.05 in the coming year, in spite of possible profit-cutting effects of removal of the new form on indomethacin from markets abroad. Although the sustained-release formula is not presently being sold in the United States, Merck has applied for FDA approval which would enable this form of Indocin to be marked domestically in the U.S..

According to Crossen, Merck will experience "long-term earning growth" of between 13 and 14 per cent. Such growth is above average compared to that in the rest of the drug industry. In Crossen's view, the growth rate may turn out to be even higher given the number of new products Merck intends to unleash on the general public over the next few years.

The Holistic Balanced Treatment is needed more than ever to bring such heinous wholesale exploitation to an end!

NAPROSYN

Naprosyn (naproxen) tablets have been advertised as anti-inflammatory in action and therefore effective in the reduction of swelling, pain and stiffness characteristic of rheumatoid arthritis. Naproxen has also been marketed as a drug able to increase joint mobility.

As indicated in the manufacturer's data sheet on Naprosyn "there is no evidence that it alters the progressive course of the underlying disease." In short, Naprosyn, like so many other drugs virtually identical to Naprosyn, treats only signs and symptoms as the underlying arthritis disease advances unchecked. Yet, even for this mere surface effect the patient can pay a high price in harmful side effects.

The safety of the drug during pregnancy and breastfeeding (lactation) has not been established so that its use is NOT RECOMMENDED for mothers-to-be or nursing mothers.

Like Indocin, Naprosyn must be administered with extreme caution to people obliged to remain alert. Naprosyn can induce DROWSINESS, DIZZINESS and DEPRESSION.

Patients receiving Naprosyn along with anticoagulants such as coumarin may develop a prolonged prothrombin time. This means bloodclotting may be seriously delayed and bleeding can result.

Naprosyn, according to Robert Mendelsohn, M.D. can also trigger life-threatening oral and rectal hemorrhaging (bleeding). One case of hemorrhaging was found to be caused by a large perforated ulcer and ruptured artery developed after Naprosyn administration.

About 14% of all Naprosyn patients develop HEART-BURN, NAUSEA, DYSPEPSIA, (stomach upset), CONSTIPATION, ABDOMINAL PAIN, DIARRHEA, VOMITING and INTERNAL BLEEDING. Skin reactions have been reported in 5% of all patients tested. These reactions included ITCHING, ERUPTIONS, ECCHYMOSES (black and blue bruises), and SWEATING. VISUAL and HEARING DISTURBANCES were also reported.

Among 737 patients treated with Naprosyn during clinical trials, 15 developed PEPTIC ULCER. Rare reactions to Naprosyn include EDEMA, JAUNDICE and THROMBOCYTOPENIA, a condition characterized by abnormally small numbers of blood platelets.

At a Congressional hearing presided over by Senator Edward M. Kennedy, FDA spokespersons indicated that

Naprosyn would never have been approved if the facts concerning its scandalously defective preliminary testing had come to light in time.

Preliminary animal testing of the drug by the Industrial Bio-Test Laboratories located in Northbrook, Illinois, did not follow accepted guidelines. Inspection of the accumulated data subsequently revealed that poor records had been kept, and that crucial mention of tumors and deaths following Naprosyn intake had frequently been omitted from the final reports!

Despite such unforgivably shoddy and unprofessional testing, the Syntex Corporation, manufacturer of Naprosyn, has been able to reap staggering profits. During the period from May to August 1976 alone, a profit of $20 million was reported!

ARALEN

CHLOROQUINE (Aralen), originally used in the treatment of malaria, has also been used for arthritis and lupus erythematosus. The danger of continued high dosages is greater than the therapeutic benefits, however.

Aralen must be utilized very cautiously in patients suffering from LIVER DISEASE, ALCOHOLISM, and BLOOD AND NERVE DISORDERS. Under no circumstances should the drug be administered to pregnant mothers or psoriasis patients.

Overdoses of Aralen have led to CARDIOVASCULAR COLLAPSE, SHOCK, CONSULSIONS and DEATH. Some of the harmful effects reported with Aralen use include HEADACHES, VISION DISTURBANCES, SKIN ERUPTIONS, NAUSEA, VOMITING, CRAMPS and DEAFNESS.

PSYCHOSES with HALLUCINATIONS as well as LOSS OF REFLEX ACTION and LOSS OF MUSCLE POTENCY IN THE LOWER EXTREMITIES can also occur. Lupus erythematosus and skin eruptions have been induced by Aralen.

Congenital deafness and retardation have been reported in the babies of mothers who took high doses of the drug during their pregnancies.

The eye injury produced by Aralen is severe and frequently irrevocable. Between 10 to 35 percent of those receiving Aralen develop deposits, on the lining of the outer coat of the eyeball called the cornea.

Changes in the retina are almost always permanent and get worse when the drug is withdrawn, Symptoms include BLURRING OF VISION and READING DISCOMFORT. More than 13 percent of all rheumatoid arthritis patients treated with chloroquin develop unwanted retinal changes.

ACTH GEL

ACTH GEL, Available only by prescription, is recommended as "adjunctive therapy" during an acute phase of psoriatic arthritis, rheumatoid arthritis, ankylosing spondylitis, bursitis or gouty arthritis.

ACTH GEL should never be administered when any of the following conditions are present: SCLERODERMA, OSTEOPOROSIS, FUNGAL INFECTIONS, RECENT SURGERY, PEPTIC ULCER, CONGESTIVE HEART FAILURE AND HYPERTENSION.

This substance can provoke hypersensitivity reactions, CATARACTS and GLAUCOMA. Not only does ACTH mask the signs of infection but it also causes new infections. The eye is one common site of such infections.

ACTH is also contraindicated for pregnant or nursing mothers since fetal defects have been reported in animals treated experimentally with the drug.

ACTH also induces HYPERTENSION, SALT RETENTION and INCREASED EXCRETION of POTASSIUM and CALCIUM.

Patients receiving the drug also should be aware that high doses obstruct antibody response which can allow infections to occur.

PENICILLAMINE

The toxicity of penicillamine, (Cuprimine, Bepen) whose mode of action in the treatment of rheumatoid arthritis is unknown, is very high. Up to 50 percent of patients are unable to continue therapy for a year. The most common reactions focus on the skin, kidney and muscle.

Several recent studies have pinpointed the hazards of penicillamine use.

A retrospective study of 156 patients (JOURNAL OF THE AMERICAN MEDICAL ASSOCIATION, October 20, 1978) yielded a high incidence of toxic reactions to the drug (62%). Reactions injurious to the kidney (nephrotoxic) were noted in 14% of patients. Seventeen patients (11%) demonstrated blood abnormalities as a result of penicillamine intake, including thrombocytopenia, a condition where there is an abnormally small number of platelets in the blood, and leukopenia, a condition where there is an abnormally small number of white blood cells.

Twenty-eight percent of patients experienced mucocutaneous toxic reactions including skin rashes, urticaria (hives), and erythema nodosum, a skin condition characterized by the formation of painful nodes in the lower extremities.

Gastrointestinal intolerance, including vomiting, nausea, cramping pain and dyspepsia, was experienced by 19 patients (12%).

According to Dr. Gary R. Epler, of the Boston University School of Medicine, penicillamine may obstruct recovery of patients suffering from such small airway diseases as bronchiolitis.

Richard G. Fischer, Pharm.D. and his colleagues in the Department of Clinical Pharmacy Practice at the University of Mississippi Medical Center, Jackson, observed acute onset of polymyositis symptoms in a 54-year-old man receiving penicillamine for rheumatoid arthritis. The polymyositis symptoms included dysphagia, swallowing difficulty, with nasal regurgitation of liquids, accompanied by dysphonia, difficulty and pain in speaking, and proximal muscle weakness.

T.J.B. Maling and C.T. Dollery of the Department of Clinical Pharmacology, Royal Postgraduate Medical School, London, England (BRITISH MEDICAL JOURNAL) have observed another complication of rheumatoid-arthritis-related penicillamine treatment: neuromyotonia. In neuromyotonia, muscles become afflicted with alternating spasm and rigidity.

Researchers at University Hospital of Wales have also observed acute colitis in a patient receiving penicillamine for rheumatoid arthritis. Colitis is inflammation of the colon.

CLINORIAL

Clinoril (sulindac) is basically a modified form of indomethacin. As pointed out by the Physicians' Desk Reference 1982, the effectiveness of Clinoril in treating patients with advanced rheumatoid arthritis has not been established.

Both PEPTIC ULCERS and GASTROINTESTINAL BLEEDING have been reported in patients taking Clinoril.

Other observed side effects include INHIBITION OF BLOOD PLATELET FUNCTION, PERIPHERAL EDEMA (swelling), HEADACHES, DIZZINESS, NERVOUSNESS, RASHES, TINNITUS (ringing in the ears), and PURITUS (itching).

A causal relationship probably does exist between Clinoril intake and the following harmful reactions: congestive heart failure in patients with extremely limited cardiac function, THROMBOCYTOPENIA, a condition in which there is an extremely limited number of platelets in the flood, LEUKOPENIA, an abnormally low level of white blood cells, VERTIGO, BLURRED VISION, and ANAPHYLAXIS, an extremely dangerous allergic reaction.

Clinoril use is not recommended for pregnant women or nursing mothers.

METHOTREXATE

According to the PHYSICIANS' DESK REFERENCE 1982, methotrexate has a "high potential toxicity".

Originally used to treat various cancers, methotrexate can produce a wide range of side-effects. Deaths have been reported following methotrexate administration in the treatment of psoriasis.

Especially at high dosages or over a long period, methotrexate is hepatotoxic (harmful to the liver) and causes LIVER ATROPHY (wasting), NECROSIS (tissue death), CIRRHOSIS, a progressive liver disease characterized by diffuse damage to liver cells, and SCARRING.

Methotrexate may also produce a conspicuous DEPRESSION OF BONE MARROW, ANEMIA, LEUKOPENIA (decreased white blood cell count), and THROMBOCYTOPENIA (reduction in the number of circulating platelets). These side effects can damage the immune system leading to infections and bleeding.

Methotrexate has caused the DEATH of FETUSES and/or CONGENITAL ABNORMALITIES, and is not recommended for women at the childbearing stage.

The most common side effects, along with LEUKOPENIA, are ULCERATIVE STOMATITIS, a mouth disease characterized by chronically recurring, painful ulcerations of the mucous lining, NAUSEA and ABDOMINAL DISTRESS.

FEVER and CHILLS, SKIN RASHES, ALOPECIA (hair loss), VOMITING, DIARRHEA, KIDNEY FAILURE, INFERTILITY, HEADACHES, DROWSINESS and CONVULSIONS are other possible side effects.

Deaths through damage to the pulmonary system (lungs) have also been reported with methotrexate use.

FELDENE

According to the Physicians' Desk Reference 1984, PEPTIC ULCERS, GASTROINTESTINAL BLEEDING and PERFORATION, piercing or tearing of the gastrointestinal tract stomach wall, have all been reported among users of the anti-arthritis drug Feldene. These side effects have sometimes been fatal.

In clinical trials involving about 2,300 patients, approximately 400 of whom were treated for over a year and 170 for over two years with Feldene, about 30% of all those receiving 20mg daily doses developed side effects. GASTROINTESTINAL SYMPTOMS were the most prevalent side effects and appeared in about 20% of patients.

In addition to gastrointestinal symptoms, EDEMA, swelling of tissues due to excessive accumulation of fluid, HEADACHES, DIZZINESS, and RASHES have been reported in some patients, as well as TINNITUS, ringing in the ears.

Decreases in hemoglobin and hematocrit, measure of proportion of red blood cells in the fluid portion of the blood indicating anemia, as well as LEUKOPENIA have also been reported with Feldene use.

As with other non-steroidal anti-inflammatory drugs (NSAIDs), Feldene-related liver function abnormalities have been noted. These abnormalities may progress or remain unchanged. The Physicians' Desk Reference does recommend that patients on Feldene with evidence of liver dysfunction should be examined for signs of more serious liver reactions during Feldene therapy.

In less than 1% of patients, the following side effects have also been observed: SWEATING, BRUISING, PHOTO-ALLERGIC SKIN REACTIONS, SWOLLEN EYES, BLURRED VISION, HYPOGLYCEMIA, WEIGHT CHANGES, DEPRESSION, INSOMNIA and NERVOUSNESS.

ORAFLEX

Oraflex was first marketed in the United States in May, 1982. It was withdrawn after a total of 12 weeks after some of its users were found to have died.

Officials at Eli Lilly and Company, manufacturers of Oraflex, have admitted that Lilly knew of 29 Oraflex-linked deaths before the drug was approved for sale in the United States on April 19, 1982.

Fraud and inaccuracy in Oraflex advertising led the Food and Drug Administration to send a "regulatory letter" to Richard D. Wood, chairman and president of the Lilly Company. Two side effects were subsequently discovered to be far more serious than the advertising campaign indicated. These side effects were a SHARP BURNING RASH affecting up to 66% of those who participated in preliminary studies of Oraflex and a condition known as onycholysis, in which the nails are loosened from their beds.

The following harmful reactions were also reported with Oraflex use: PEPTIC ULCER, GASTROINTESTINAL BLEEDING, HEART PALPITATIONS, DEPRESSION, CONFUSION, PINPOINT HEMORRHAGES (PETECHIAE), ANEMIA, HYPERTENSION, HEART FAILURE, TINNITUS (TINGING IN THE EARS), VISION DISTURBANCES, HEARING LOSS, HEADACHES, VERTIGO (DIZZINESS), SLEEP DISTURBANCE and DRYNESS OF EYE and MOUTH.

Chapter IV
The Case Against Surgery

More than two million unnecessary surgical operations, including hysterectomies, tonsillectomies, appendectomies and coronary bypasses were performed in 1977, according to a report by the House Subcommittee on Oversight and Investigations of the parent committee on Interstate and Foreign Commerce.

Representative Douglas Walgren, member of the subcommittee, considers that 17 percent of all hospital operations are not needed. Other subcommittee officials believe that patients should always obtain second and even third opinions before undergoing surgery of any kind.

If the physician giving the second opinion is a surgeon, he or she should always be a **salaried** staff surgeon rather than one who is paid for the operation. The probability of a tonsillectomy being performed on a Blue Cross subscriber is about four times as great as for a **prepaid** health plan subscriber.

THE IMPORTANCE OF THE HOSPITAL CHOICE

It has been noted that surgical risks vary from hospital to hospital, Dr. Crile of the House Subcommittee on Oversight has urged that each hospital publish mortality rates for every type of operation so that patients can be made aware of risks **in advance.**

Dr. Crile has also urged that surgery be done in large medical centers rather than small institutions. For example, in large centers, coronary bypass operations are a standard procedure. In most small institutions, coronary bypass operations are performed very infrequently. As a result, the risks are much greater — ten times as great, in fact.

DANGER OF SURGERY FOR DAMAGED JOINTS

According to Dr. William H. Harris of the Department of Orthopedic Surgery, Massachusetts General Hospital (NEW ENGLAND JOURNAL OF MEDICINE) joint replacement surgery can produce a wide range of post-surgical complications.

Total hip replacement surgery, for example, is linked to a relatively high incidence of thromboembolic disease. A thrombus is a clot formed in a blood vessel or one of the cavities of the heart.

The incidence of thromboembolic disease after total hip replacement is 50 percent.

Another danger of joint replacement surgery is infection. Deep infections can occur as late as eight years after the operation. In most cases, infection is introduced by bacteria at the time of the operation.

In most cases when a total hip replacement becomes infected, the implant must be removed. The patient then has a flail hip. One leg is necessarily shorter than the other and a built-up shoe, crutches and canes become necessary.

The replacement of other joints in the body involve even greater risks than replacement of the hip joint.

For example, failure rates of up to 25 percent are typical in the first three years after **total knee replacement.** This can be explained, in part, by the fact that the knee is a highly complex joint because of the structural intricacies of the ligaments that underpin knee stability.

The **total elbow replacements** attempted in the 1970's have been almost total failures.

When administered early enough, the Holistic Balanced Treatment eliminates the need for joint replacement surgery by stimulating the body to heal itself.

However, if joints are injured to such a degree that surgery becomes necessary, then this dynamic threefold approach — balanced hormone medication, diet and exercise as able — optimally prepares the body for a shorter convalescence and a minimum of surgical complications.

Chapter V
The Holistic Balanced Treatment For Arthritis Diseases

T he Holistic Balanced treatment, a dramatically innovative threefold approach to arthritis, has been administered successfully to over 30,000 patients without life-threatening side effects.

Unfortunately, there are still millions of Americans suffering from the various forms of arthritis disease — rheumatoid arthritis, osteoarthritis, ankylosing spondylitis, juvenile rheumatoid arthritis and gouty arthritis — who have not been alerted to the availability of the Holistic Balanced Treatment.

Too many of these arthritis sufferers have come to depend on ultimately useless painkillers with severe side effects such as aspirin, Butazolidin, Motrin, Indocin, Naprosyn, Clinoril, and penicillamine.

As drug manufacturers candidly admit, these products do nothing to confront the underlying arthritis disease. Over time, larger and larger dosages must be used to mask pain for shorter and shorter intervals as the disease process advances unchecked.

Restoration of a positive protein-building balance is crucial for both healing of tissue injured by arthritis and ongoing optimum lifelong health.

Robert Liefmann, M.D., who developed the Holistic Balanced Treatment over several decades of extensive research in Mexico, Scandinavia and Canada, discovered that the correct combination of hormones naturally found in the body — in this case, prednisone, testosterone and estradiol — could restore the protein-building balance while at the same time stopping arthritis pain and inflammation. Hormones, produced by specialized body organs known as glands, regulate and control a vast array of vital processes in the body, including growth, breathing, and the breakdown of proteins, sugars, starches and fats for use by body cells.

ADDITIONAL BENEFITS OF THE HOLISTIC BALANCED MEDICATION

The Holistic Balanced medication is never administered without considering the particular needs of the individual patient. The medication is adjusted for every patient on the active roster so that the proper tissue-building and healing response can be obtained. Respect for the uniqueness and the unique needs of the individual patient is one of the essential principles of the holistic approach to health.

In sharp contrast to the other drugs for arthritis, the Holistic Balanced medication does not encourage an evergrowing dependence on larger and larger dosages. In fact, smaller quantities of the Holistic Balanced medication have consistently been found, in time, to be as effective as initial larger amounts. In cases where the arthritis has been brought under control and symptoms completely eliminated, the medication may no longer be necessary.

DIET AND EXERCISE

Proper diet is crucial for the healing of tissue injured by arthritis and for the prevention of unwanted flare-ups of the disease, as well as for general good health.

The person receiving the Holistic Balanced Treatment

plays an active role in creating and maintaining a diet which harmonizes with these worthy aims. Taking personal responsibility for one's own fitness and well-being is, we might add, another cornerstone of the holistic approach to health.

The unique components of the Holistic Balanced diet are explained and described at length in the HOLISTIC DIET AND COOKBOOK, published in an attractive soft-cover edition by the Institute for Research of Rheumatic Diseases and available at an equally attractive low price (see page 00 for details).

We can only summarize the key points here.

The Holistic Balanced diet emphasizes fresh fruits and vegetables, sunflower seeds, raw unsalted high-protein nuts, such as cashews, peanuts, almonds and English walnuts, pure health food store peanut butter, 100% whole grain breads, noodles, cereals and pastas, foods high in calcium such as milk, cheddar cheese, bran, spinach and beets, protein-rich organ meats, soy beans, dried peas and organic eggs. For drinking, distilled, spring or mineral water as well as herbal caffeine-free teas, Pero and Postum, are recommended.

THE WRONG KIND OF DIET AND ITS CONNECTION WITH DISEASE

In addition to flare-ups of arthritis, scientific evidence has shown that the wrong kind of diet has been associated with heart disease, cancer, diabetes, obesity, and dental problems.

The wrong kind of diet is typically high in: 1) sugar and sugar products, i.e. candy, ice cream, soda, jams, cakes, chewing gum, 2) salt and foods spiced and cured with salt, such as luncheon meats and a wide variety of canned foods, 3) empty-caloried processed foods such as those containing white flour and hydrogenated or partially hydrogenated fats, found, for example, in margarine, solid vegetable shortenings and commercial peanut butter, and 4) coffee, tea, alcohol, and tobacco.

The Holistic Balanced diet urges the complete elimination of these disease-producing dietary components and is able to suggest healthful and savory substitutes for all of them. For example, frozen apple juice concentrate, apple juice or apple cider can be substituted for sugar in cooking.

When uncontrolled, arthritis causes destruction of cartilage, muscle and bone, disfigurement and crippling. It may even spread to organs outside initially affected joints, such as the skin, nerves, heart and lungs.

People with arthritis who take these drugs quickly find themselves in a state of serious physical, emotional and financial dependency. Such dependency, affecting millions, insures drug companies their staggeringly large profits.

Limited — almost nonexistent — effectiveness must be measured against the often life-threatening side effects of these drugs. Butazolidin and Tandearil have both been linked to leukemia. Motrin is associated with dangerous blood disorders. Aspirin interferes with bloodclotting and the body's utilization of vital vitamin C, and may produce gastrointestinal bleeding and ulcers.

According to Roland Moskowitz, M.D., Professor of Medicine, Case Western Reserve University, Cleveland, Ohio, aspirin intake has been found to cause hepatitis and to impair kidney function.

Clinorial can cause peptic ulcers, ringing in the ears (tinnitus), visual disturbances and emotional depression.

Oraflex — removed from the market in August 1982 after a brief run — was found to cause fatal liver and kidney damage.

WHAT MAKES THE HOLISTIC BALANCED
TREATMENT DIFFERENT FROM ALL THESE DRUGS

Unlike all other drugs and approaches presently available, the Holistic Balanced Treatment is a **complete** treatment for arthritis.

A complete treatment not only stops pain and inflammation but also grapples effectively with the underlying disease process to prevent irreversible crippling and deformity.

The Holistic Balanced Treatment — which consists of a balanced hormone medication, sound diet and exercise and activity as able — confronts and ultimately triumphs over the underlying arthritis disease by restoring the positive protein-and-tissue-building balance upset by the bodily stress of arthritis.

EXERCISE AND ACTIVITY

Exercise and physical activity are vital to the healing of arthritis-damaged tisue, as well as the prevention of crippling and deformity and the restoration of physical movement.

In THE LANCET, a magazine for physicians, a British researcher has recently shown how regular exercise can help prevent fractures in postmenopausal women with osteoporosis and may actually contribute to an increase in bone mass.

As with medication and diet, exercise is geared to the unique and changing needs of the individual patient.

As painful symptoms begin to disappear, patients are encouraged to engage in gentle stretching, deep abdominal breathing, and non-strenuous swimming, as well as normal walking around the house. Good posture enhances the benefits that may be derived from these activities.

When the arthritis is under control and painful inflammatory symptoms (stiffness, soreness, tenderness) are completely eliminated, patients may progress to more demanding stretching and straightening exercises for specific joints.

HOPES FOR THE FUTURE AND FOR THE MILLIONS OF ARTHRITIS SUFFERERS

Every arthritis sufferer has a right to know that there is a viable alternative to ineffective life-threatening painkillers.

Every arthritis sufferer has a right to know that this alternative, available now, permits the resumption of a much more normal, fulfilling and active life than could ever be possible with aspirin, Clinoril, penicillamine, Naprosyn or Motrin.

Every arthritis sufferer has a right to know that because of the Holistic Balanced Treatment — the only viable alternative— arthritis need no longer be thought of as an overwhelming and hopeless handicap that must be passively accepted along with splints, crutches, canes and wheelchairs.

Chapter VI
The Holistic Approach To Health And Well-Being

*H*olism, or holistic healing, is clearly an important concept whose time has come.

The strength of the concept of holistic healing can be evaluated both by the continuing dramatic effectiveness of the Holistic Balanced Treatment for crippling arthritis diseases, and by the ever-growing interest shown by "orthodox" medical practitioners in this invaluable and unique approach to medical care.

As pointed out by Malcolm C. Todd, M.D. ("Interface: Holistic Health and Traditional Medicine", WESTERN JOURNAL OF MEDICINE), the word "holistic" derives from the Greek "holos" meaning whole.

Holistic healing may therefore be defined as that approach to health which emphasizes and seeks to ensure unification of mind, body and spirit in the person being treated.

Over 2,000 years ago, the pioneering Greek physician Hippocrates insisted that the whole person must be taken into account if medical problems are to be resolved properly. The whole person is affected not only by the life processes occurring within the body but also by changes in the social and physical environment.

DISSATISFACTION WITH TRADITIONAL
HEALTH CARE DELIVERY

What accounts for the widespread dissatisfaction with "orthodox" scientific medicine, hospitals and health care in the United States?

The present system of conventional medical care focuses more on diagnosis and treatment of existing illness and less on **prevention** of illness with accompanying encouragement of over-all good health.

In contrast, holistic health concentrates on personal well-being as a strenuous commitment. Just how healthy we are ultimately depends on how much active responsibility we are willing to assume in our pursuit of health.

The interdependence of mind, body and spirit is one of the axioms of holistic medicine. Dr. Herbert Benson, director of the behavioral medicine division of Beth Israel Hospital in Boston and faculty member of the Harvard Medical School, has devoted over ten years to studying how mind affects body.

THE MIND/BODY CONNECTION AND
MEDITATION TECHNIQUES

According to Dr. Benson, our response to environmental stressors is accompanied by increased use of oxygen, accelerated heart rate and raised blood pressure (hypertension).

Dr. Benson's investigations led him to the practice of transcendental meditation. He found that meditation could reduce both oxygen consumption and respiration rate, as well as the blood lactate levels associated with anxiety and hypertension.

The Boston physician and his colleagues have identified 4 components of transcendental meditation: 1) sitting quietly 2) closing the eyes 3) repetition of a word or phrase compatible with the meditator's beliefs and 4) dismissal of any other thought that may enter the mind.

This form of relaxation has been highly effective in treating abnormal heart rhythms, pain, and anxiety, and is one of many examples of how a serious commitment to mental and spiritual well-being can alleviate and reverse harmful **body** changes.

THE HOLISTIC PRACTITIONER ALSO USES
TRADITIONAL CONCEPTS AND TECHNIQUES

It is important to remember that holistic health is a **fusion** of traditional medical concepts and techniques and the fundamental principles of the holistic approach.

The holistic physician is simply much more attuned to the other factors — physiological, biochemical, genetic, nutritional, environmental, psychological and immunological — at work in health and disease.

CONCRETE EXAMPLES OF THE HOLISTIC APPROACH

In his essay, "Holistic Health: A Valuable Approach to Medical Care" (WESTERN JOURNAL OF MEDICINE), Marc Lappe, Ph.D., Acting Director of the Hazard Alert System of the California Department of Health Services at Berkeley, discusses the holistic perspective as an invaluable tool for understanding specific diseases such as arthritis.

Recent advances in arthritis research suggest that many factors, besides bacterial infection and the wear-and-tear of aging, such as immune reactions and heredity may interact to set arthritis in motion. There may very well be no single cause of arthritis but rather many that unite to produce the disease.

Recent advances in immunology and genetics have revealed what holistic practitioners have long known — there are dramatic differences in the biochemical make-up of individuals. Physicians administering the Holistic Balanced Treatment take this fact into consideration at all times by gearing the medication to the changing needs of the individual patient. Diet and exercise are similarly adjusted and developed to meet the needs of the individual patient.

HOLISTIC THINKING AND
ANKYLOSING SPONDYLITIS

Genes transmit information crucial for survival from parent to offspring. A good example of a special kind of gene is HLA-B27, which has been linked to ankylosing spondylitis. This form of arthritis disease in which the spine is bent permanently forward as the spinal bones (vertebrae) fuse has been successfully treated by the Holistic Balanced Treatment. The correlation between this particular gene and the appearance of ankylosing spondylitis has been carefully charted by P.I. Terasaki (NEW ENGLAND JOURNAL OF MEDICINE.)

More than 95 percent of all young men who develop ankylosing spondylitis possess this gene. However, the sole presence of this factor is not sufficient to induce the onset of ankylosing spondylitis, because less than 2 percent of all people with HLA-B27 become afflicted. Emotional or physical stress, or contamination with certain distinct bacterial species, may also play a role.

It is the holistic perspective — with its emphasis on the subtle interweaving of many factors to produce the uniqueness of each individual — that has helped give researchers a clearer idea of the causes of diseases like ankylosing spondylitis.

Chapter VII

Scientific Support And Experimental Studies Show The Holistic Balanced Treatment Works

*A*t about the same time that Dr. Robert Liefmann was developing the Holistic Balanced Treatment in Canada, medical researchers in the United States were utilizing a balanced combination of hormones in the treatment of rheumatoid arthritis and related arthritis conditions.

Dr. Philip Hench, 1950 winner of the Nobel Prize in physiology and medicine, was one of the pioneers in the field of balanced hormone research.

When Dr. Hench and his colleagues treated rheumatoid arthritis with cortisone alone ("Effects of Cortisone Acetate and Pituitary ACTH on Rheumatoid Arthritis, Rheumatic Fever and Certain Other Conditions, A Study in Clinical", ARCHIVES OF INTERNAL MEDICINE, Volume 85, Number 4, April 1950), they observed many unwanted side effects from exclusive use of the drug. When cortisone was combined with testosterone and estradiol, utilization of the three hormones in balance led to almost total abolition of these unwanted side-effects.

In another study by Hench and his colleagues, estrone (estradiol, estrone and estriol are three variants of the female sex hormone estrogen), and progesterone were administered before and during cortisone therapy, after a broad spectrum of side effects had resulted from cortisone therapy alone. The utilization of the three hormones (estrone, cortisone and testosterone) led to total abolition of not only menopausal symptoms but of almost all other side effects as well. These side effects included rounding of the face, breathing difficulty, nervous tension, mild hirsutism, headaches and globus, or the sensation of compression in the throat. The efficacy of estrone was further confirmed by partial recurrence of some of these symptoms once use of the female sex hormone was discontinued and cortisone alone therapy resumed.

Dr. William Ishmael and his colleagues at the University of Oklahoma School of Medicine ("Effects of Certain Steriod Compounds on Various Manifestations of Rheumatoid Arthritis," JOURNAL OF THE OKLAHOMA STATE MEDICAL ASSOCIATION, October, 1949) also carried out research furnishing remarkable corroboration for Dr. Liefmann's own work.

The Oklahoma researchers observed 90 patients treated with compounds of testosterone and estradiol over a one to three month interval. Four of the patients failed to respond to the balanced hormone treatment and five underwent irregular periods of remission.

At the commencement of treatment, many of the patients had irregular cycles of remission and flare-up but, when the proper balance between the hormones was refined, the number of patients responding unpredictably was reduced to five out of 90 patients.

Dr. Ishamel diagnosed a participating patient as being in

remission when he or she was free of pain, swelling, and morning stiffness, had a normal appetite, and was not anemic. On the basis of these criteria, 81 patients were found to have gone into remission as a result of the balanced hormone medication administered.

As a more refined balance between the hormones was achieved, the unwanted side effects of testosterone and estradiol were eliminated. Pregnenolone, a steriod hormone, was subsequently added to the testosterone-estradiol mixture. Testosterone, the researchers found, was most effective in controlling rheumatoid arthritis symptoms, as well as inducing better appetite and sleeping habits.

A more recent study in support of balanced hormone therapy for arthritis was performed by Harold Varon, M.D., James Finney, Ph.D. and Robert Millwee, M.D. of Baylor University, Dallas, Texas, ("New Treatment for Rheumatoid Arthritis Using Sex Hormones", presented at the Southern Medical Association's 69th Annual Scientific Meeting, Miami Beach, Florida, November 16-19, 1975).

In their study, Dr. Varon and his colleagues evaluated the responses of 14 women with severe rheumatoid arthritis to the hormones estrogen and progesterone. These hormones were used in quantities comparable to those generated during pregnancy.

Varon, Finney and Millwee based their rheumatoid arthritis treatment approach on the work of Dr. Philip Hench. In 1938, Dr. Hench observed the effect of 34 pregnancies on 20 women with rheumatoid arthritis. Thirty out of 34 pregnancies produced considerable or total relief from the inflammatory symptoms of rheumatoid arthritis. Later, Dr. Hench and his colleagues observed a total of 150 rheumatoid arthritis patients. The majority of these exhibited significant or total improvement during their pregnancies. ("The Potential Reversibility of Rheumatoid Arthritis", Abstract of the Heberden Oration, delivered before London's Heberden Society, October 5, 1948).

The 14 women who participated in the Varon study ranged in age from 39 to 61, and suffered from rheumatoid arthritis for six to twenty-three years. They received complete physical examinations, along with laboratory tests of complete blood count, urinalysis, sedimentation rate to evaluate extent of inflammation, SMAC 20 chemistries, and endocrine (gland function) studies.

Treatment during the experiment consisted of large weekly doses of estradiol cypionate, progesterone in oil, and medroxyprogesterone acetate, injected intramuscularly. Response to the hormones occurred within a few days time and was frequently very marked. Decrease in joint pain and swelling was accompanied by increased range of movement and physical strength. Moreover, there were no recurrences of inflammatory joint swellings.

Preliminary laboratory testing indicated moderate to severe joint involvement in most of the patient subjects. After the balanced hormone treatment, sedimentation rates diminished and six of the fourteen patients exhibited normal sedimentation rates indicating the inflammation was thoroughly under control. Before commencing treatment, 12 of the patients exhibited moderate anemia; after treatment, all 12 had hemoglobin levels situated in the normal range.

X-ray studies after balanced hormone treatment revealed a lessening of both soft tissue swelling and osteoporotic (bone softening and thinning) changes. Radiological studies also demonstrated increase bone calcification indicating a corresponding increase in bone density.

Dr. Varon and his colleagues observed a marked improvement in emotional and mental outlook among all those treated with the balanced hormone medication.

In addition to the corroborative results derived from these studies, the Physician's Desk Reference also furnishes support for utilization of a balance of hormones in arthritis disease therapy.

According to the PDR, Estratest is a useful adjunct in long-term corticosteriod therapy. Estratest contains both esterified estrogens and testosterone, in the form of methyltestosterone. Among the positive benefits of Estratest are an ability to alleviate bone pain and assist in stopping the catabolic (breakdown) process in osteoporosis.

THE EXPERIMENTAL STUDY OF DR. LIEFMANN

Dr. Robert Liefmann evaluated the effect of the Holistic Balanced Treatment through a controlled scientific study.

The effect of the Holistic Balanced Treatment on rheumatoid arthritis in relation to disease activity, laboratory changes, side effects in general emotional and mental well-being, was evaluated in 373 patients.

These 373 patients, who ranged in age from 3½ to 103 years, were distributed geographically over the United States and Canada. The number of male patients was approximately equal to the number of females.

During the study, a sound and simple diet was followed by the subjects. The diet encouraged protein, and natural starches and sugars from fresh fruits and vegetables. Processed sugar was eliminated and in some cases animal fat consumption was restricted. Supplements included such vitamins and minerals as bone meal, vitamin C, vitamin B complex, natural vitamin E and potassium. These supplements were prescribed as indicated by individual needs.

The study used the subjects as their own controls. Therefore, there was no additional group of subjects in which one of the crucial experimental conditions was omitted for purposes of comparison. Before treatment, the arthritis disease status of each subject was evaluated over a daily three-day period in order to establish a definitive level of affliction.

The measurements carried out on the subjects included blood and urine studies and joint function analysis. The latter was determined by such parameters as degree of pain, degree of swelling, amount of heat and range of movement in the joints.

In a second three-day period, all the patients were given placebos and the same measurements were repeated. A placebo is a substance with no known physiological effect. Instead, it may have a suggestive effect on the recipient.

The placebo period was followed by administration of the Holistic Balanced medication along with the carefully formulated diet. Measurement of disease activity through laboratory tests and joint function analysis continued. Neither the nurses administering the medication nor the doctors evaluating the patients knew whether placebo or Holistic Balanced medication was being administered. A study in which neither the patient nor the organizers know what kind of medication is being given at a specific time is called a "double-blind."

In all subjects, joint pain, swelling and stiffness had persisted throughout the evaluation period and during the period of placebo administration. After the Holistic Balanced Treatment was begun, however, the disease process in each patient was stopped and functional improvement commenced.

Before Treatment, 77% of the subjects had continuous pain; 44% were afflicted with deformities; 37% were disabled; 76% experienced swelling; 42% reported feelings of weakness; and 36% had indigestion.

Also before Treatment, 49% of the subjects suffered from impairment in activity. In this category were patients obliged to use wheelchairs, canes, braces, crutches, or splints, as well as semi-bed patients.

After the Holistic Balanced Treatment began, pain relief was distributed as follows:

PAIN RELIEF AFTER START OF
HOLISTIC BALANCED MEDICATION

Elapsed time	Number of subjects experiencing relief
12 hours or less	109
13-24 hours	76
1-2 days	30
3-7 days	29
8-14 days	12

130 patients were eventually able to walk without support and 143 experienced much improvement in their range of activity.

Of the 373 patients originally participating in the Liefmann study, 55 (or 15%) eventually went into complete remission — they no longer required medication. The 220 patients (59%) who did without the medication all experienced a gradual relapse of their arthritis disease.

Many of the original 373 patients, along with approximately 7,000 others, remained on the Holistic Balanced Treatment for a 14-year follow-up period. During this follow-up period, physicians well-versed with all aspects of the Holistic Balanced Treatment found no clinical or laboratory evidence of gastrointestinal ulcers, osteoporotic changes (in which bones become brittle, fragile, less dense) or nitrogen depletion. Reported side effects were remarkably few and could always be consigned to the category of minor and reversible nuisances.

Over the 14-year period, patients experienced good results in the restoration of joint movement and tissue healing with smaller doses of the Holistic Balanced medication. The dosages selected for patients based on unique individual need were frequently deminished to very small maintenance dosages.

RHEUMATOID ARTHRITIS

Mrs. Cynthia Clemente
11301 175 Road, North Jupiter Florida 33458

Mrs. Cynthia Clemente experienced rheumatoid arthritis symptoms for the first time in 1972 at the age of 19.

Initially, the arthritis was limited to her jaw and elbows. Over a two-and-a-half year period during which time she was under the care of a conventional arthritis doctor, the arthritis spread to all regions of her body, except her knees and hips. She was unable to turn her head.

The medication she was taking included 30 aspirin tablets day and caused headaches, ulcers and ringing in the ears (tinnitus).

Just before beginning the Holistic Balanced Treatment when her arthritis was at its most excruciating, Mrs. Clemente found herself spending approximately $1000 per month on pain-killers. Her doctor admitted that he could not offer any other help and suggested that she enter a crippled children's center in Palm Beach.

On May 25, 1977, the morning after her first Holistic Balanced Treatment, Mrs. Clemente awoke with virtually no pain. Before the Treatment it used to take her a half-hour to get out of bed.

Three days later, feelings of soreness and stiffness were also gone.

At present, Mrs. Clemente is pain-free and works out three times a week at a health spa.

She continues to take the Holistic Balanced medication, a flare-up occurred once when she forgot to take it, but at present her dosages are much smaller then they were initially.

RHEUMATOID ARTHRITIS

Mrs. June Mills
9240 Lantern Road, Lake Worth, Florida 33463

Mrs. Mills developed symptoms of rheumatoid arthritis in 1977, at the age of 49.

Over a two-year period, she received gold injections, pencillamine, small amounts of prednisone in tablet form, Butazolidin, and sixteen aspirin tablets a day, as well as other medications.

Her medication cost averaged about $100 per week.

None of the medications were of any use. However, they were all her Palm Beach County-based rheumatologist could offer.

Before receiving the Holistic Balanced Treatment, Mrs. Mills hands and shoulders were immobilized and she could not turn her head. In addition, her liver and kidneys had deteriorated and her stomach was seriously injured.

She wondered if there was any point in living under these circumstances.

She was obliged to give up her privately-owned business as a certified hearing aid audiologist because she simply could not work. Her medical bills were ruinous.

Against the strong advice of her physician, Mrs. Mills decided to receive the Holistic Balanced Treatment. Reports from five patients, two men and three women, already receiving the Holistic Balanced Treatment were extremely favorable and encouraging.

Mrs. Mills' pain was gone the second morning after she received her first Holistic Balanced Treatment in July 1979. She woke up able to move ankles, hands and feet. Her arthritis improved steadily and within two months she was no longer aware that she had rheumatoid arthritis.

She began using a bicycle, dancing and going to the beach. Before receiving the Holistic Balanced medication she had been unable to get up once she lay down in the sand.

With her arthritis presently under control, Mrs. Mills has reduced her medication by more than half her starting dosage.

RHEUMATOID ARTHRITIS

Malcolm Simmons
37 Morris Drive, Hyde Park, New York 12538

Mr. Malcolm Simmons had his first attack of arthritis in 1936, at the age of 21. The pain became constant in 1959. Deformities were first noticed in 1960. Involved were his shoulders, hips, knees, upper and lower spine and breast bone. At that time, his knee condition was being aggravated by his work of plumbing and heating installation as he had to kneel on rough surfaces.

In 1954, he had severe iritis (inflammation of the eyes) frequently seen in Rheumatoid Arthritis. In June, 1961, extensive retinal hemorrhages were found in both eyes.

From 1961 to July, 1962 Mr. Simmons tood 12-14 tablets of aspirin daily. From May, 1961 to June, 1962 he received cortisone injections in his right knee once a week. Dolcin was prescribed by his physician without relief. He applied liniments and, following his doctor's advice, tried to keep moving.

He began this treatment on August 1962 after reading a May 1962 *Look* magazine article. He experienced dramatic and enduring relief of his symptoms.

According to his physician, Henry Little, M.D., "his arthritis had almost disappeared and his eyes were normal." The change immediately after the Balanced Hormone Treatment was "most dramatic." He had been like an old man with his arthritis.

Unable to obtain medication in 1968, symptoms including retinal hemorrhages and iritis began returning. He again had complete relief after taking this hormone medication again.

51

RHEUMATOID ARTHRITIS

A. Glenn Manon
1698 Streator Avenue, Washington, Pennsylvania 15301

Mr. Glenn Manon had his first manifestations of arthritis in 1956 with slight occasional pain.

Constant pain began in 1961 in shoulders, elbows, wrists, knees, ankles, all ten fingers, and upper spine.

Before beginning treatment on September 17, 1973, he usually took 14 aspirin tablets per day, as prescribed by his physician with different types of diet, dry and wet heat treatments, and liniments.

Twenty four hours after his first Holistic Balanced Treatment, Mr. Manon experienced significant relief of his pain, swelling and stiffness of hands, wrists, elbows, feet, knees. This improvement continues throughout the treatment and after.

RHEUMATOID ARTHRITIS

Carolyn Sue Marley
4115 Langden Road, Winston Salem, North Carolina 27107

Mrs. Marley had had vague arthritis complaints since her high school years. In 1964, at the age of 27, she was diagnosed as having Rheumatoid Arthritis. The disease process began in the knees and spread to all joints except the spine, though there was occasional cervical (neck) stiffness.

Deformities, though minimal, were first noticed in 1970. In 1971, synovectomy operationson both knees were done.

From July 23, 1973 until August 26, 1976, she received biweekly gold injections as prescribed by her physician with Indocin, aspirin, cortisone, heat treatments and liniments for her deteriorating condition. Her body ached and her joints remained stiffly impaired, deformities were increasing with weakness, indigestion, nausea and lack of appetite.

Four hours after taking this treatment, on October 13, 1976, she had almost complete relief of her pain. Swelling and stiffness were also dramatically reduced. Her strength returned. She had been a semi-bedpatient requiring splints. She has since been capable of performing all her regular activities.

RHEUMATOID AND OSTEOARTHRITIS

Mr. William Murphy
3107 Huntington Street, Orlando, Florida 32803

Mr. Murphy began the Holistic Balanced Treatment on March 26, 1976. He had suffered from the aches and pains of Rheumatoid Arthritis for many years. In September, 1975, the pain became constant and his activity was greatly limited. In 1976, deformities were evident in shoulders, wrists, knees and fingers.

He had received cortisone injections in the left knee and shoulders. He took prednisone in tablet form for ten days in 1976. Indocin caused stomach problems. Deformities of hands and knees increased with generalized weakness and lack of appetite.

He had severe pain in hands, shoulders, knees and feet. Six hours after taking this treatment, he had significant relief of the severe swelling in knees and complete relief of swelling of his hands.

He continues to feel fine, with knee, elbows and shoulder joints all greatly improved and confirmed by laboratory findings.

JUVENILE RHEUMATOID ARTHRITIS

P.R.
Willingboro, New Jersey

P.R. first had arthritis in 1963, in the shoulders, elbows, wrists, hips, knees, jaw and fingers, at age six. He had two hip replacement operations at the University of Pennsylvania Graduate Hospitals in 1975 and wrist and finger synovectomies between the ages of eight and nine. At age 12 he had surgery on both knees.

After beginning the Holistic Balanced Treatment on October 3, 1974, he had relief of pain, stiffness, weakness and swelling in his joints. He has continued to improve dramatically. He even had an increase in growth. After the treatment, he was able to continue and complete school studies previously interrupted.

RHEUMATOID ARTHRITIS

Dr. Thomas M.
Sunnyvale, California

Dr. Thomas M. first had arthritis in 1968, at the age of 39. Pain became constant in 1975 and the following year deformities were noticed in the left shoulder, right elbows, both wrists, right knee, both ankles, upper spine, jaw, all ten fingers and all toes. He subsequently became disabled.

A local physician precribed aspirin in 1975, diet, heat and professional physical therapy with no improvement whatsoever.

Dr. M. first heard about the Holistic Balanced Treatment through his doctor and a friend. A day after his first Holistic Balanced Treatment, on April 27, 1977, he was able to close his fist and wear shoes for the first time since January of that year. He is now able to lift furniture whereas before he had not been able to lift the telephone.

LETTERS
Some Examples

I would like to shout to the entire world about what if has done for me. I had been on cortisone and gold injections for four years and was in so much pain I couldn't turn over in bed or sit up without help. My knees down to my big toe were swelled huge. I couldn't spread my toast because I could not use my hands at all. I couldn't feed myself because I couldn't raise my arms. I sat like this in a hospital bed. . .for four and a half months. I had been to doctors here and also in Phoenix, Arizona, with no relief.

My niece then took me to Montreal to see Dr. Liefmann. I got the medicine, and I took three doses from 1 p.m. until 10 p.m. About 12:00 I told my niece I felt the swelling leaving and she didn't believe it. The next morning. . .I drove home, 800 miles from Montreal. I haven't been disabled since. I bake and decorate cakes again. I have no side effects of any kind and wish everyone who has arthritis could get this medicine.

Get this medicine on the market so all sufferers can have

access to it. Without it I would be a complete cripple; with it, I am once again a useful person.

Mrs. La-Reta Hoover
Rural Route 5, Box 339
Edwardsburg, Michigan 49112

I have been on this medicine for a long time since October 15, 1974. As far as I am concerned it gave me a chance to life my life like a normal human being. Neither I nor my family have regretted by decision to go on it.

Mrs. Audrey Champney
Route 1
Colton, New York 13625

I wake up in a brand new world every day. I think I am enjoying life more now than ever before. Thank you for giving me a second shot at living. I feel like it's better than the first. No way can I express my gratitude to you and your staff for my health and happiness.

Mr. Tom Crosslin
Route 8, Box 69C

I would like to mention that my arthritis was diagnosed as Pierre-Marie Strumpel spondylitis. This is the type that bends the patient double. In August 1962 when I started the medication, I weighed 149 pounds and was using a cane. I could not turn my head and could do no physical work. Today I weigh 190 pounds (I am 5'11"), show absolutely no sign of arthritis, and maintain an active schedule seven days a week. I have had my blood checked three times and each time, I have been pronounced to be in top physical condition.

I would like to add that in 1961 I was in a hospital for tests and observation. X-rays showed that by hips were so clouded with calcium that the joints could not be seen and five vertebrae in my back were fused. I was told that in about five years I would be so bent that I would not be able to sit in a wheelchair. About five years ago, for my own information, I had a set of X-rays taken and was told that my back and hips were in better condition than the average person's.

Mr. Malcolm Simmons
37 Morris Drive
Hyde Park, New York 12538

It has been a source of great satisfaction and encouragement being a patient with your clinic. For the first time in 35 years I feel that I am receiving effective treatment from professionals who not only have an understanding of all facets of the disease but have empathy with the patient.

Fannie Henderson
Box 67
High River, Alberta, Canada TOL1BO
Sparta, Tennessee 38538

March 14, 1979
To: Arthritis Medical Center,
I came to the Arthritis Medical Center directly from Toledo Hospital in Toledo, Ohio, where I had spent 27 days with eight doctors on my case. These were four Rheumatologists, a Neurosurgeon, Neurologist, Internist and an Orthopedic Surgeon. They said there was nothing more they could do for me.

Upon entering Arthritis Medical Center, I was unable to move even a finger. I weighed 63 pounds and had no control of my kidneys. Sixteen hours after taking medication from the clinic I was able to move my fingers, and from that time forward there has been a steady improvement. I can now walk and use my hands and now weigh 97 pounds. Mr previous average weight was approximately 100 pounds. I lived a relatively normal life after eight months on the medication and am still improving.

I thank God that I was directed to the Arthritis Clinic and wish that all the people who are afflicted with this painful disease had the opportunity to visit this clinic.

Katherine Wagoner
205 Andover Place
Sun City Center, Florida 33570

Chapter VIII

The Holistic Balanced Treatment And Establishment Medicine

Regressive medical bureaucracies dedicate a substantial part of their energy and industry to snuffing out the exciting discoveries of independent medical researchers. At this very moment a medical breakthrough is probably being bypassed simply because it was made outside the pale and without the dubious blessings of bureauratized establishment medicine.

The career of Dr. Robert Liefmann, developer of the Holistic Balanced Treatment for arthritis diseases, illustrates all too vividly the problems and frustrations of the truly creative medical researcher harassed and hounded by an envious and inert medical monolith.

The Holistic Balanced Treatment was developed during decades of extensive research in Mexico at the Benjamin Franklin Library in Mexico City, in Sweden at the Sudsjukuset Hospital and Southern Hospital, both in Stockholm, and in Canada at the Royal Victoria Hospital. Intensive research culminated in the publication of his discoveries in the prestigious Swedish medical journal Acta Medica Scandinavica. Dr. Liefmann also treated many arthritis sufferers with dramatic success both in Mexico and Sweden before establishing his own arthritis practice in Montreal, Canada.

Dr. Liefmann was guided by the principle which states that the stress of arthritis disease causes a hormone imbalance in the person with arthritis.. By recreating the correct combination of hormones in quantities analogous to those found **naturally** in the body, Dr. Liefmann was able to restore the balance necessary for the healing of arthritis-injured tissue and optimum lifelong health.

The hormones used by Dr. Liefmann were prednisone, a hormone with anti-inflammatory properties; testosterone, a protein-building sex hormone; and estradiol, a protein-building female sex hormone. However, Dr. Liefmann brought his combination of hormones to a very high level of refinement and therapeutic efficacy before providing his treatment to patients.

Before his death in October, 1973, Dr. Liefmann experienced difficulty with the Food and Drug Administration in Canada. FDA agents posing as needy arthritis patients, requested an interim supply of the medication from his secretary until an appointment could be made. As a result of these officials' dishonesty, Dr. Liefmann found himself prosecuted for violation of the Food and Drug Act that prohibits the selling of medication to people who are not patients. Dr. Liefmann as a phisician, could combine approved drugs for his patients only.

On countless occasions, Dr. Liefmann had generously offered his arthritis medication to the Canadian government, and showed himself consistently willing to share his discoveries with his colleagues. Unfortunately the Food and Drug Administration, along with regressive physicians, were unmoved by such a display of dedication. The FDA and the medical community were united by a single aim: the destruction of Robert Liefmann and his work.

Finding himself cornered, Dr. Liefmann called upon Professor Henry B. Rothblatt, the distinguished American criminal attorney, to assist the Canadian lawyers already defending him. Many of Dr. Liefmann's grateful patients attested with fervor to the astonishing effectiveness of his approach — the only one which had allowed them to resume relatively normal and fulfilling lives. Only mere technical violations of the law were proven. There was absolutely no evidence of criminal wrong-doing.

The matter was settled and Dr. Liefmann continued to practice medicine and relieve arthritis suffering.

The difficulties resurfaced, however, when, after Dr. Liefmann's untimely death, the Holistic Balanced Treatment began to be administered at offices in New York City and in Florida. In response to attempts by the Arthritis Foundation, Escambia County Medical Society and the Attorney General of Florida to obstruct utilization of the Holistic Balanced Treatment, Professor Rothblatt demonstrated that over 30,000 patients had been safely treated over a 25-year period and, once again as in Canada, that all components of the medication — prednisone, estradiol and testosterone — were FDA-approved substances. The Arthritis Foundation and the government and medical groups unscrupulously allied against the Arthritis Medical Center and Arthritis Medical Offices were obliged to concede, before a federal judge, that its staff had a perfectly legal right to administer their treatment.

Why has the Canadian and American FDA both, along with the medical establishment, exhibited such strong hostility toward the Holistic Balanced Treatment? Greed and the prospect of enormous profits play a crucial role in this hostility.

Drug companies are only interested in drugs for which they can ultimately obtain an exclusive patent. These corporate giants exert a powerful influence on both the FDA and the medical establishment through the staggeringly liberal monetary favors they are always willing to bestow in pursuit of their central aim — profit.

The ingredients of the Holistic Balanced medication are readily available. Therefore, drug companies have consistently shown no interest in this medication. They will undertake a multimillion-dollar testing program only if there is a substantial prospect of an exclusive patent. The FDA and medical establishment, driven by their deep-rooted dependencey on the drug companies and by their own jealous rage at authentic medical innovation, show the same mixture of indifference and envy toward the Holistic Balanced Treatment.

As long as it exists, this dynamic threefold approach poses a very real threat to profit-hungry drug companies and medical practitioners. When the Holistic Balanced Treatment becomes as widely known and accepted as its success with over 30,000 patients indicates that it very much deserves to be, then all other arthritis drugs and provisional treatments will disappear.

Dr. Liefmann was never interested in profit. His concerns lay elsewhere in bringing genuine relief to the person suffering from arthritis. Physicians skilled in administering the Holistic Balanced Treatment in New York City and in Fort Lauderdale, Florida, wholeheartedly share his vision.

Chapter IX
The Positive Benefits Of Estrogen

*E*strogen in the form of estradiol is one of the three hormones which contribute to the dramatic effectiveness of the Holistic Balanced medication.

Estrogen, the female sex hormone, and testosterone, the male sex hormone, are both anabolic. This means that they work to restore the body's positive tissue and protein building balance upset by arthritis.

Estrogen, secreted by the ovaries, is responsible for the development of sexual characteristics.

During a woman's reproductive years, estrogen causes thickening of the uterine lining. This thickening prepares the uterus for possible reception of a fertilized egg.

At the time of menopause, estrogen production either becomes minimal or ceases completely. Twenty-five to thirty-five percent of all women experience acute symptoms during menopause. These symptoms include hot flashes, sweating, chills, depression, fatigue and diffuse anxiety. Osteoporosis, or bone thinning, may also become a serious problem for some women, causing fractures and pain.

For women who develop these symptoms, estrogen therapy can inaugurate a return to general well-being and increase of energy.

61

ESTROGEN AND CANCER

Dr. Robert Greenblatt, professor emeritus of endocrinology at the Medical College of Georgia at Augusta, has been prescribing estrogen therapy for over 35 years. Dr. Greenblatt has encountered only five cancer cases out of the 1,000 women examined each year over that thirty-five year period. He warns physicians against easy intimidation by reports of increased cancer risk among estrogen users.

Dr. Robert W. Kistner of Harvard Medical School in Cambridge, Massachusetts, has been prescribing estrogen for twenty-five years, and has seen only five cases of cancer among his menopausal patients. These five, according to Dr. Kistner, failed to follow clearly defined therapeutic guidelines.

Dr. Lila Nachtigall and her colleagues at New York University have studied the long-term effects of estrogen therapy. Twelve years ago, they divided 168 female subjects into two groups. The 84 participants in the first group took daily estrogen along with another female hormone progesterone, one week out of every month. The other 84 participants received placebos — substances which have no known medical effect on the patient. They may, however, exert a suggestive effect.

The results of the Nachtigall study show that the fear of cancer among estrogen users may be unwarranted. Not one case of cancer among the hormone users was reported. However, there was one case of uterine cancer and four cases of breast cancer among the placebo-takers.

ESTROGEN PROTECTION AGAINST OVARIAN CANCER

According to a four-year study conducted at the Boston University School of Medicine Drug Epidemiology Unit (FLORIDA NURSING NEWS), women who use oral contraceptives are half as likely to contract ovarian cancer as other women.

The results of the study suggest that estrogen-containing oral contraceptives furnish protection against this form of cancer which may last for as long as a decade.

ESTROGEN AND THE BREAST CANCER RISK

According to Dr. R. Don Gambrell and his colleagues in the department of obstetrics and gynecology at the Welford Hall U.S. Air Force Medical Center (MEDICAL TRIBUNE), postmenopausal women receiving estrogen therapy have a lower risk of developing breast cancer than women who have never received estrogen therapy.

In their study, Dr. Gambrell and his colleagues examined 5,263 postmenopausal women in the period of 1975-78. The women examined were either Air Force employees or dependents of Air Force employees.

The incidence of breast cancer among women never treated with estrogens or oral contraceptives was much higher 441 per 100,000, than the incidence of breast cancer among women who received estrogen therapy. Breast cancer incidence among those who received estrogen was much lower — 142 per 100,000. The difference in incidence is, in Dr. Gambrell's view, statistically significant.

Apart from lower incidence of breast cancer, women receiving estrogens who did develop breast cancer had a better prognosis, or forecast of disease outcome, than women who had never received estrogens. Only 15.2 percent of the patients who developed breast cancer during estrogen therapy died. In contrast 34 percent of the women who developed breast cancer without ever having received estrogens died. This difference is of statistical significance.

In Dr. Gambrell's view, the Wilfred Hall study supports other studies demonstrating no enhanced risk of breast cancer from estrogen therapy. In addition, studies such as the Third National Cancer Survey show no correlation between oral contraceptives and breast cancer.

MENOPAUSAL ESTROGEN THERAPY AND PROTECTION FROM DEATH FROM ISCHEMIC HEART DISEASE

A study by Ronald K. Ross, Thomas M. Mack, Annlia Paganini-Hill, Mary Arthur and Brian Henderson ("Menopausal Estrogen Therapy and Protection from Death from Ischemic

Heart Disease," THE LANCET, April 18, 1981) suggests that estrogen replacement therapy in postmenopausal women may protect against death from ischemic heart disease, in which the blood supply to the heart becomes obstructed.

ESTROGEN AND OSTEOPOROSIS

Estrogen has been shown to be highly effective in the treatment of osteoporosis and bone loss in women. Osteoporosis is a condition of increased porosity and fragility of bone due to a reduction in the quantity (mass) of bone. According to MEDICAL TRIBUNE, most of the 200,000 fractures that are sustained annually occur among women with osteoporosis. In addition to causing great suffering, these fractures represent an $800 million annual expense for the nation.

There is a lack of evidence that estrogen treatment can prevent fractures. However, for the approximately 7.5 million women with a milder degree of bone demineralization, there is much greater hope. Estrogen treatment may enable them to retain a significant amount of bone mass.

SCIENTIFIC SUPPORT FOR
ESTROGEN THERAPY IN OSTEOPOROSIS

One important study has come from Omaha, Nebraska's Creighton University. Dr. Robert P. Heaney, professor of internal medicine and vice-president of health sciences, and Dr. Robert R. Recker, associate professor of internal medicine and director of the Bone Research Unit, supervised a study of 60 healthy Catholic nuns between the ages of 55 and 65. These subjects received a balanced dosage of estrogen and testosterone 21 days a month over a two-year period. A second group received calcium. A third group served as controls.

The results were obtained through exquisitely precise X-ray measurements. These results showed that bone mass in the controls decreased 1.18% per year as compared to 0.15% in the balanced hormone group and 0.22% in the calcium group.

The rate of decrease in bone mass was therefore eight times as great in the control group without calcium or estrogen as compared to the balanced hormone (estrogen and testosterone) group!

Dr. Joseph Picchi, clinical professor of internal medicine at the University of California, has been co-researcher in one of the longest estrogen-osteoporosis studies ever made. About 220 women with osteoporosis and vertebral fractures received daily estrogen, skipping only the first 5 to 7 days of the menstrual cycle, from 1948 to 1955. About 12 of these women are still receiving the estrogen therapy.

According to Dr. Picchi, decrease in bone density has been minimal and all those who followed carefully-defined guidelines report no fractures. These guidelines included a balanced diet and moderate activity.

THE LEEDS STUDY

Dr. Christopher Nordin and his colleagues at the Mineral Metabolism Unit of the General Infirmary, Leeds, England, have also carried out a study for the treatment of osteoporosis. Dividing 82 women averaging 62 years of age with fragile bones into 6 groups, the Leeds researchers went on to measure their progress utilizing several different clinical parameters. Most of the women participating in the study were followed for at least 2 years.

Dr. Nordin found that estrogen used in combination with either two specially-activated forms of vitamin D was the most effective therapy for osteoporosis. The other therapies used were ranked in decreasing order of efficacy: calcium supplements, estrogen alone, ordinary vitamin D and calcium, only one of the specially-activated forms of vitamin D,and ordinary vitamin D alone.

Dr. Nordin defined "efficacy" as the capacity to arrest loss of bone. In estrogen-vitamin D therapy he actually detected a small bone-density gain.

The Leeds group presented its findings at an International Symposium on Osteoporosis in Miami, Florida. The researchers gathered there were particularly impressed by the wide variety of methods through which Dr. Nordin and his colleagues measured the effectiveness of the therapies tested. These methods included x-ray, measurement of bone resorption (loss) through radioactive tagging of calcium, measurement of height loss, and counting of vertebral compression fractures.

During 10 years of experience prescribing estrogen, Dr. Nordin has not encountered a single case of endometrial cancer.

OTHER STUDIES

A study by Claus Christiansen, Merete Sanvig Christensen and Ib Transbol ("Bone Mass in Postmenopausal Women After Withdrawal of Estrogen/Gestagen Replacement Therapy", THE LANCET, February 28, 1981), has investigated the effect of estrogen on the amount of bone after menopause and, particularly, on the rate of bone loss after estrogen therapy ended.

Over a three-year period, ninety-four healthy female volunteers who previously passed their natural menopause six months to three years ago, participated in the study.

Christiansen and his colleagues found a significant and continued increase in the amount of bone during the three-year estrogen therapy. The quantity of bone was 8 percent higher in the ninety-four women who received estrogen therapy, than in those who received no estrogen.

Results with women who discontinued estrogen therapy during the study period suggest that EVEN TEMPORARY ESTROGEN THERAPY WILL HAVE A LASTING BENEFICIAL EFFECT ON THE QUANTITY OF BONE.

REDUCED RISK OF HIP AND LOWER FOREARM FRACTURES WITH POSTMENOPAUSAL ESTROGEN USE

The most frequent sites of fracture among many postmenopausal women are the spinal bones, forearm and hip.

A study by N.S. Weiss, M.D. and his colleagues at the University of Washington ("Decreased Risk of Fractures of the Hip and Lower Forearm with Postmenopausal Use of Estrogen," THE NEW ENGLAND JOURNAL OF MEDICINE) found that the risk of fracture to the hip or forearm was fifty to sixty percent lower in women who used estrogens for six years or more, than in women who had not used them.

Clearly, estrogen and hormone treatment is an invaluable therapeutic tool when used properly. Such therapy has a great deal to offer in a wide range of conditions, including osteoporosis, with little or no medical risk.

Chapter X

Clarifying The Many Misconceptions Regarding The Holistic Balanced Treatment

Over the years, the Holistic Balanced Treatment for arthritis diseases has been the target of many misconceptions and rumors, as well as the outright vicious slander of journalists and "hired guns".

Many people put great faith in the authority of the FDA. According to Dr. Sidney Wolfe, director of the Public Citizen Health Research Group located in Washington, D.C., and affiliated with Ralph Nader — one of the great crusaders for the rights of the consumer against profit-hungry industry — the FDA has been unable to fulfill its promise to the people.

Pat McGrady, Sr., medical editor for the MEDICAL TRIBUNE and author of THE PERSECUTED DRUG, recently demonstrated how FDA cowardice and ignorance have resulted in unpardonable delays in approving the drug DMSO. Highly refined scientific research indicates that DMSO is capable of a wide range of therapeutic effects which haven't even begun to be scruitnized by the drug industry and regressive members of the medical establishment.

A REVEALING STUDY

A three-year study by the General Accounting Office of the United States Government (MEDICAL TRIBUNE) has revealed that the FDA is staggeringly inefficient in evaluating new drug applications. Of 132 drug applications submitted in 1975, only 69 were approved after a four-year period. With regard to fourteen important drugs, the study disclosed that thirteen were available in Europe up to thirteen years before they were even approved in the United States.

Some groups defend the slowness of the FDA in making decisions as proof of this bureaucracy's delicate alertness to the risks involved and passionate concern for patient safety.

We do not agree. When a patient stands between life and death and a lifesaving drug is available, the FDA has no right to prevent this drug from being administered. What matters most is a patient's health and safety AT THE MOMENT WHEN THAT PATIENT REQUIRES EFFECTIVE CARE.

THE ARTHRITIS FOUNDATION

Despite its much-praised efforts, the Arthritis Foundation has only approved aspirin and its many variants as effective therapies against arthritis. The side effects — biochemical, physical, financial — of aspirin are devastating and we will be discussing them in depth. Generous endowments from the drug companies are given to the Arthritis Foundation.

We might mention the postgraduate seminar on management of arthritis held by the Arthritis Foundation in association with Blue Cross Blue Shield Insurance Company in St. Augustine, Florida, November 12-14, 1981.

The purpose of the seminar was to educate physicians about current drugs and surgery for arthritis. Administered early enough, the Holistic Balanced Treatment eliminated the need for surgery, as well as the crutches, splints, canes, wheelchairs and other health aids advocated by the Arthritis Foundation.

What is especially revealing is the fact that the seminar committee acknowledged the support of the following drug companies in making the seminar possible: McNeil Laboratories, which manufactures Tolectin for arthritis, Merck, Sharp and Dohme, penicillamine, Sulindac, indomethacin, Parke-Davis aspirin, Syntex Corporation, Naprosyn, Upjohn Company, aspirin, cortisone, Ibuprofen, and Dista Company, manufacturers of Nalfon.

The interconnections do not stop here. These products basically camouflage the underlying arthritis disease but produce enormous profits for the drug companies. Yet, all the products were listed as arthritis "therapies of choice" in the September, 1980 FDA CONSUMER, along with surgery, heat, splints, crutches and braces.

NO MEDICATION FOR ARTHRITIS HAS JUSTIFIED ITS CLAIMS MORE THOROUGHLY THAN THE HOLISTIC BALANCED TREATMENT. In other chapters, we deal with the long research tradition that culminated in the Holistic Balanced Treatment and the many short- and long-term research studies that establish Holistic Balanced Treatment's effectiveness.

According to Dr. Sidney Wolfe, drug companies can falsify their results with ease if they wish.

Over the past ten years, Industrial Bio-Test Laboratories (IBT) near Chicago, Illinois, has carried out more than 22,000 scientific testing projects on chemicals and drugs, including the arthritis drug Naprosyn. About 50 percent of these research studies were used to obtain government approval for the products tested.

In May, 1981, after a five-year FDA-U.S. Department of Justice Investigation, the president of IBT and three of his colleagues were indicted by a federal grand jury in Chicago. They were charged with performing fake scientific research and with distributing fake data supposedly based on that research.

In a crucial section of the final report on Naprosyn, manufactured bySyntex Corporation, IBT furnished false blood and urine data. According to the government, IBT's claim that it performed complete autopsies and thorough microscopic studies of test animals treated with the arthritis drug was also false!

Here we have an example of the FDA participating in the unearthing of a fraud.

The relation between Burton, Parsons and Company, a Maryland company producing solutions to clean contact lenses, and two FDA regulators has been under Congressional investigation.

The question examined by the Oversight and Investigations subcommittee of the House Committee on Energy and Commerce was whether the wining and dining of two FDA experts by the management of Burton-Parsons led to its gaining A MONOPOLY OVER PRODUCTS IN ITS FIELD.

The Congressional subcommittee has released detailed expense account vouchers showing how Burton-Parsons officials paid for dinners and repeated trips to the racetrack for the two FDA officials, who were entertained lavishly not only in the nation's capital but also in New York, New Orleans, Las Vegas and Paris!

Entertainment expenses totalled $9,000 over a five-year period, during which time an FDA ban on alternative lens-cleaning products, less-expensive salt tablets, was instituted. The ban made Burton-Parsons the primary if not the only supplier of FDA-approved lens-cleaning products.

FELDENE

Since April of 1982, the anti-arthritis drug Feldene, manufactured by Pfizer, Inc., has been prescribed to over 1 million people suffering from the disease. Feldene has also been prescribed to more than 10 million foreign patients with arthritis.

FDA documents and official testimony before the House of Representatives intergovernmental relations subcommittee indicate Feldene causes VERY SERIOUS SIDE EFFECTS, such as intestinal bleeding and ulcers.

When Feldene was in the testing stage, Pfizer chose to administer the drug to arthritis patients already using aspirin and other products like aspirin. When the FDA's Bureau of Drugs finally got around to warning Pfizer that simultaneous use of aspirin in testing represented a weighty flaw, the testing process had already been concluded.

At first, Pfizer's application for Feldene was rejected by the FDA. A subsequent reassessment proved equally disturbing and revealed striking inconsistencies in Pfizer's claims for its drugs.

Pfizer research studies indicated that Feldene could relieve symptoms of osteoarthritis, the most frequently encountered form of arthritis. Unfortunately for Pfizer, one of the FDA statisticians participating in the reassessment found that:

1) Some of the patients in the studies had been examined by completely different investigators, making it extremely difficult to disentangle the data and pinpoint individual conditions.

2) There were many mysterious corrections and changes overwritten on the study reports.

3) In one study, one-third of the patients were not suffering from osteoarthritis at all!

In spite of heated debate among FDA staff members regarding the flagrant inadequacy of the data available on Feldene, Dr. Marion Finkle, head of new drug evaluation, decided to grant FDA approval to the drug.

ORAFLEX: ANOTHER ARTHRITIS DRUG

Oraflex, developed by Eli Lilly and Company, was marketed in the United States for a total of 12 weeks before being withdrawn in August 1982 after some of its users died.

During that 12-week period, approximately 500,000 patients obtained prescriptions for Oraflex from their doctors.

In contrast to Pfizer — which focused on falsifying its rudimentary research data on Feldene — Eli Lilly and Company succeeded in painting a very pretty picture of Oraflex through advertising, promotional pamphlets and press kits.

ORAFLEX AND THE WORLD OF ADVERTISING

Drug companies have customarily publicized prescription drugs only among private physicians. However, because no law actively forbids advertising among patients, many companies have started to reach out to the patient population through news releases and television. As Lawrence K. Altman, M.D. (THE DOCTOR'S WORLD: "Oraflex Promotion Produced Sales But Not Without Side Effects": NEW YORK TIMES) points out, drug companies commonly spend tens of millions of dollars on their advertising stratagems and ploys.

THE CASE AGAINST ZOMAX

In early March, 1983, Zomax, a drug manufactured by Johnson and Johnson, was abruptly withdrawn from drugstore shelves. The withdrawal of the drug, a nonsteroidal anti-inflammatory agent like Oraflex, followed widely publicized news reports indicating that Zomax caused **allergic reactions** in some patients. Johnson and Johnson then admitted that these allergic reactions resulted in five deaths since marketing of Zomax had begun two years before.

However, until the adverse reactions and deaths were made public (WALL STREET JOURNAL, Tuesday, March 8, 1983), there was never any indication that Johnson and Johnson intended to pull Zomax out of circulation.

This reluctance may be related to the fact that, according to the New York Times (March 9, 1983), worldwide sales of Zomax during 1982 amounted to 83 million dollars. Johnson and Johnson reaped a profit of 60 million in the United States alone!

THE HOLISTIC BALANCED TREATMENT: WHAT SETS IT APART FROM ALL OTHER APPROACHES

The Holistic Balanced Treatment, by restoring the positive protein-building balance distrubed by the stress of arthritis, permits healing of disease-injured tissue. This ability to assist and stimulate tissue healing through restoration of positive balance distinguishes the Holistic Balanced Treatment from all other treatments. Treatments such as aspirin, gold, cortisone, Clinoril, Feldene, penicillamine, Naprosyn, and indomethacin, merely mask symptoms of pain and inflammation as the under-lying arthritis progresses unchecked to cause disfigurement, deformity and crippling.

Physicians skilled in administering the Holistic Balanced

Treatment are the first to admit that prednisone, one of the components of the medication, when **used alone,** does lead to the breakdown of body tissue. However, all charges laid at the door of prednisone are rendered meaningless in the case of the Holistic Balanced Treatment. This approach utilizes a balance of hormones — testosterone and estradiol, both tissue building (anabolic) sex hormones — to counteract and completely cancel the destructive side effect of prednisone when combined with prednisone in the appropriate amounts.

Interference with resistance to infection has not been seen in over 22 years experience administering the Holistic Balanced Treatment. Over this period of time, 30,000 patients have been successfully treated.

The few side effects that do occur with administration of the Holistic Balanced Treatment are minor nuisances that are rapidly brought under control.

Although prednisone alone may trigger the development of stomach ulcers, there has been no incidence of stomach ulcers with the Holistic Balanced Treatment. As we have already pointed out the Treatment is a carefully compounded mixture of testosterone, estradiol and prednisone.

According to the **British Medical Journal,** however, steroids alone may not be implicated in the development of stomach ulcers. An analysis of 42 double-blind controlled trials of steriods in the treatment of a variety of diseases — including rheumatoid arthritis — has shown NO DIFFERENCE in the incidence of dyspepsia or gastrointestinal hemorrhage between active and placebo groups.

In studies where a history of peptic ulcer was common, there was NO EVIDENCE OF REACTIVATION IN THE GROUP TAKING STEROIDS. These data are consistent with experimental evidence that steroids do not increase occult gastrointestinal blood loss or cause gastric erosions.

The British Medical Journal article was the work of P.L. Zentler-Munro and T.C. Northfield of the Department of Medicine, St. George's Hospital Medical School, London, England.

SIDE EFFECTS OF ASPIRIN

In contrast to the Holistic Balanced Treatment, aspirin and its variants produces a wide range of unwanted side effects. Aspirin can cause internal bleeding, stomach ulcers and vitamin C depletion.

According to the HARVARD MEDICAL SCHOOL HEALTH LETTER, five percent of all cases of terminal kidney disease in America may have their roots in excessive intake of pain relievers such as aspirin.

The Holistic Balanced Treatment is NOT A CURE for arthritis. Given the present state of our medical knowledge concerning arthritis, the Holistic Balanced Treatment is simply the only effective treatment available now.

Physicians informed of the astonishing effectiveness of the Holistic Balanced Treatment are always eager to work with patients' local doctors. Many local doctors dedicated to the well-being of their patients, have referred their patients to the Arthritis Medical Center.

ROLE OF DIET

Proper nutrition is an important component of the Holistic Balanced Treatment.

An article appeared in MEDICAL WORLD NEWS indicating that arthritis symptoms could be provoked by the intake of certain foods. Dr. Marshall Mandell, medical director of the Alan Mandell Center for Bio-Ecologic Diseases, conducted a study of forty patients with arthritis complaints and subjected them to diverse food extract and chemical allergens. The results of the study were reported to the American College of Allergists at a congress in Bal Harbor, Florida. Dr. Mandell found that joint and muscle pain, depression, headache, fatigue, confustion and bowel and bladder problems could be produced in response to intake of such foods as soybean, sugar, milk, coffee and egg.

Dr. Mandell's work is just one example of a growing awareness on the part of the hither-to-backward medical community regarding the close connection between diet and disease flare-ups.

Each day brings new research indicating how improper diet can lead to cancer, heart disease, diabetes, arthritis, and dental disorders. Similarly, there are independent studies that confirm how a proper diet, plentiful in fresh fruits and vegetables, nuts, seeds, calcium-rich products, unfluoridated water, 100% whole grains, and organic eggs, can prolong life and guaranteed biochemical, mental and emotional well-being.

The Holistic Balanced Treatment, combining medication, diet and exercise as able has been in the vanguard of this trend through its insistence on the role of extra medicinal factors in maintaining overall good health.

Chapter XI

Nutrition: Vital Component Of The Holistic Balanced Treatment

Proper nutrition, based on a sound diet emphasizing natural foods, is vital to the healing of arthritis-injured tissue as well as lifelong good health and well-being.

The Holistic Balanced diet emphasizes fresh fruits and vegetables; high-protein nuts and seeds; some meat, fish, fowl, cheese, organic eggs; 100% whole grain breads, cereals, pasta; and, fluoride-free distilled, spring or mineral water.

Sugar and sugar-containing products, such as, candy, ice cream, soda, jellies, cakes, pies and chewing gum; empty-caloried processed and "junk" foods; fried foods; salt and foods cured or spiced with salt such as, luncheon meats, soft cheese, canned vegetables, soups and stews; hydrogenated or partially hydrogenated fats found in margarine, solid vegetable shortenings and most commercial peanut butters; and coffee, tea, alcohol and tobacco, all alarmingly increase the risk of heart disease, cancer, diabetes, arthritis, obesity, and dental disorders. All these products are eliminated from the Holistic Balanced diet and healthful substitutes found wherever possible.

For example, frozen apple juice concentrate, apple juice or apple cider are excellent replacements for sugar in cooking. Uncooked fats, butter, cream, mayonnaise, sugar-free salad dressings and cold processed vegetable oils such as sunflower and corn oils, can always be used in place of cooked or hydrogenated fats to make meals savory and energy-packed. Herbal teas and coffee substitutes such as Pero and Postum are very good hot beverages which may be used in place of caffeine-laden drinks. Caffeine provides the body with the wrong kind of stimulation. Coffee drinking, we might add, has been linked to pancreatic cancer.

There are a wide range of natural flavorings, herbs, and spices which may be used in place of salt. Green pepper, fresh lemon juice, marjoram, fresh mushrooms, parsley, sage and thyme enhance the flavor of chicken. Bay leaves, green peppers, lemon juice, marjoram and fresh mushrooms all go well with fish. Chives, garlic, dill, onion, parsley, basil and oregano can all be used with various vegetables.

CALCIUM

Calcium is a mineral needed by every part of the body. Calcium is essential to heal damaged joints. In combination with phosphorus and vitamin E, calcium builds bones and teeth. Calcium also assists in bloodclotting and is vital for the proper functioning of muscle, nerve and heart tissue.

According to D.L. Scott and his colleagues ("Serum Calcium Levels in Rheumatoid Arthritis", ANNALS OF THE RHEUMATIC DISEASES), blood calcium levels in people with rheumatoid arthritis are lower than in healthy subjects. When blood calcium levels are low, and insufficient quantities are obtained from the diet, the body must obtain this important mineral from storage centers located in the bones and teeth. The consequent calcium drain can cause the development of brittle porous bones which fracture easily. This condition is known as osteoporosis.

77

According to Dr. David A. McCarron, kidney specialist at the University of Oregon Health Sciences Center (NATURAL HEALTH BULLETIN) calcium deficiency may also cause hypertension (high blood pressure). A diet plentiful in calcium and very low in salt might therefore be considered a potent stabilizing influence on blood pressure.

Substantial evidence indicates that calcium can be highly effective in relieving anxiety, nervousness, irritability, tension and fear. This is because calcium is able to bind with lactate (lactic acid), a normal by-product of our body processes, according to Dr. John Wozny, of the Department of Educational Psychology of the University of Alberta, Canada (NERVES, EMOTIONS AND YOUR HEALTH, Rodale Press).

High calcium foods include milk, cheese (specifically the cheddar type), apricots, cabbage, cauliflower, celery, spinach, beets, bran, raw organic egg yolk, lemons, onions, cranberries, radishes, Swiss chard, string beans, endives, cucumbers, broccoli, soy-beans and kale.

Calcium is also available in health food/vitamin stores, in the form of egg shell tablets, oyster shell tablets, powdered or tablet bone meal, calcium gluconate, calcium orotate, calcium lactate and chelated calcium. It is a good idea to try different forms.

ANOTHER VITAL MINERAL

Potasium is needed to strengthen skeletal and internal muscles, and to prevent digestive disorders. The person with arthritis has a special need for supplementary sources of potassium to restore levels depleted by the arthritis.

Natural sources of potassium include bananas, corn, apple peel, dandeloin, watercress, lima beans, red beets, parsley, cabbage, broccoli, peaches, celery, cucumbers, eggplant, green peppers, parsnips, rhubarb, spinach, romaine lettuce, Swiss chard, 100% whole wheat, tomatoes, asparagus and grapefruit juice.

FOCUS ON VITAMINS

Vitamin A deficiency can produce symptoms of burning and itching in the eyes, night blindness, acne, lack of appetite and disorders in fat storage and the dry mucous linings of the mouth, respiratory system and genitourinary system. Vitamin A, a potent protector against colds and pneumonia, combats infection by strengthening those mucous linings susceptible to germ infiltration.

According to Dr. Richard Doll, president of the British Association for Cancer Research (HEALTH CARE NEWS), there is a relationship between a reduced risk of lung cancer and the vitamin A found in carrots. His most recent research indicates a 40% lower risk of developing lung cancer in experimental animals receiving carrots in their diet compared to animals receiving no carrots.

A study by Dr. Saxon Graham and his colleagues at the State University of Buffalo and Roswell Park Memorial Institute (THERAPAEIA Magazine) suggests that vitamin A and vitamin C in the diet may reduce the risk of laryngeal cancer.

Clearly, the positive effect of vitamin A intake on potential cancers is an extremely fertile area for research.

Good vitamin A sources include apricots, broccoli, carrots, cheddar cheese, Swiss cheese, organic eggs, cod liver oil, cream butter, milk, lettuce, prunes, spinach, peppers, tomatoes, cantaloupe, nectarines, peaches and pumpkin.

THE WIDE SPECTRUM OF B VITAMIN ACTIVITY

The B vitamins are necessary for overall good health. Irritability, depression, skin problems, poor appetite, anemia and constipation can all occur because of vitamin B deficiency.

Thiamine or vitamin B_1 has a beneficial effect on the nervous system, mental outlook and learning ability. It is also necessary for normal growth in childhood and improvement of muscle tone in the heart and gastrointestinal tract.

Common early signs of thiamine deficiency include constant fatigue, lack of energy, inability to sleep or eat well, crossness and irritability. According to Miriam E. Lowenberg (FOOD AND MAN, John Wiley and Sons), dietary lack of thiamine may not be great enough to cause illness but may nevertheless produce noticeable symptoms.

Alterations in mood may be the first sign that thiamine is lacking. If this sign is heeded potentially permanent changes in the brain can be prevented.

Other signs of thiamine deficiency include faulty memory, concentration, emotional instability and overreactions to the stresses of everyday life.

In Dr. Lowenberg's view, brown rice and cereal grains are fine sources of thiamine. Neither white flour nor white rice have appreciable levels of thiamine because the vitamin is found in the germ and outer coatings of cereal. These valuable nutrient sources are discarded in the refining process.

Vitamin B_2, or riboflavin, is involved in the metabolism of nutrients such as carbohydrates (sugar and starches) and proteins. It is also necessary for good vision, skin and hair.

Good riboflavin sources are organ meats. Try to avoid animal liver or kidney. These organs filter the many toxic materials of our environment.

Dr. William Kaufman, in his book "The Common Form of Joint Dysfunction: Its Incidence and Treatment", has shown that vitamin B_3, or niacin, has a positive effect on arthritis. After administering large doses of niacin to patients with significant joint dysfunction, Dr. Kaufman noted remarkable benefit to afflicted joints.

Dr. Roger Williams, author of "Nutrition Against Disease" refers to the results of Dr. Kaufman's study that found injured joint cells are somehow prevented from receiving an adequate supply of niacin. Large supplemental doses of this vitamin somehow insure that an adequate supply reaches the cells.

Wheat germ, Brewer's yeast, lean meats, poultry, fish and peanuts are rich sources of niacin.

Pantothenic acid, manufactured in the body by friendly bacteria residing in the intestines, is another important member of the B-vitamin group. Brewer's yeast, organic egg yolks, 100% whole grain cereals and organ meats are the most plentiful sources of pantothenic acid.

This vitamin is useful in treating arthritis. According to a British study (LANCET) blood levels of pantothenic acid in people with arthritis are lower than those of healthy subjects. The severity of the disease may also be correlated with pantothenic acid levels. When pantothenic acid was administered to participants in the study, relief of arthritis was immediate.

A LOOK AT VITAMIN B₆

Dr. John Ellis, author of "The Doctor Who Looks At Hands" has been treating arthritics with vitamin B_6 for many years and has found it effective in relieving pain, stiffness and the "locking" of finger joints.

Daily doses of vitamin B_6 have also been found successful in relieving the pains and discomforts produced by birth control pills, pregnancy and menstruation.

Dr. Gideon Seaman, director of medical education at Creedmoor Psychiatric Center in New York, considers vitamin B_6 one of the safest substances a woman can take to achieve total or partial relief from pregnancy-related symptoms of breast pain and nausea.

Premenstrual tension, menstrual cramps and the acne flare-ups that occasionally accompany menstruation may all be dramatically reduced through vitamin B_6 intake.

Organ meats and whole grains, as well as Brewer's yeast are the best sources of this vitamin.

VITAMIN C

Vitamin C enhances resistance to infection, assists in the healing of broken bones and wounds, helps prevent tooth decay and soft gums, and improves absorption of vital minerals.

Vitamin C also prevents tiredness and loss of appetite, and helps guard against excessive or abnormal bruising.

According to Dr. Roswell R. Pfister, chairman of the department of ophthalmology at the University of Alabama Eye Foundation Hospital, vitamin C is very effective in preventing perforation and ulceration in the corneas of eyes. The cornea of the eye is a transparent lining found in the outer coat of the eyeball. Preservation of the cornea can make the difference between seeing and not seeing.

Highly successful results with animals have led to large scale clinical trials of vitamin C in treating human eye burns.

VITAMIN C AND CANCER

Drs. William F. Benedict and Peter A. Jones of Children's Hospital in Los Angeles, California (MEDICAL TRIBUNE), have found that low doses of vitamin C can prevent or cancel the changes in living cells which normally occur after these cells are exposed to carcinogens.

Along the same lines, Dr. John H. Weisburger of the American Health Foundation (MEDICAL TRIBUNE) believes the significant drop in stomach cancer in the United States over the last forty years may be due to the presence of vitamin C in lettuce and other vegetables.

Dr. Weisburger's population and laboratory studies suggest that the vitamin C in vegetables prevents the formation of cancer-causing substances in the body. These carcinogenic substances are often derived from the nitrites found in luncheon meats, pickled fish and mackerel.

Adding to vitamin C's impressive array of disease-preventing credits is its capacity, along with calcium, to protect against heart disease specifically ischemic heart disease, in which the blood supply to the heart is somehow defective. This capacity to protect against heart disease was revealed in a British study by E.G. Knox (LANCET) through autopsy measurements. Canadian researcher G.C. Willis (JOURNAL OF THE CANADIAN MEDICAL ASSOCIATION) has found that the lowest levels of vitamin C are often present in those deceased subjects whose heart disease was most serious and of longest duration.

Good sources of vitamin C include citrus fruits, tomatoes, green peppers, broccoli, raw greens, cabbage and potatoes.

A NOTE OF SELENIUM

Selenium is a mineral found in the soil and in various foods. Recent studies suggest that selenium deficiency can produce a wide range of emotional and physical ailments.

An impressive body of evidence demonstrates that cancer deaths are more prevalent in regions where the soil levels of selenium are low.

According to Dr. Gerhard N. Schrauzer, professor of chemistry at the University of California in San Diego, selenium may also help prevent heart disease. Statistics indicate that the higher the blood selenium levels in a given cross section of the population, the lower the death rate from heart disease.

Reduced bruising and increased healing have also been helped with selenium.

Selenium can be obtained in your local health food store.

Good dietary sources of this versatile mineral include 100% whole wheat bread, fresh fish, garlic, asparagus, seaweed, raw unsalted nuts, seeds, apricots, organ meats and yeast.

COOKING HINTS

Extremely valuable cooking hints and techniques for healthful preparation of foods, as well as a wide variety of tasty, easy-to-follow recipes are available in the HOLISTIC DIET AND COOKBOOK, published by the Institute for Research of Rheumatic Diseases. This book demonstrates how the guiding principles of the Holistic Balanced diet can be dynamically put into practice for good health, long life, and exciting culinary experiences.

APPENDIX: PRODUCTS TO AVOID

SUGAR

In addition to being one of the major culprits in the genesis of heart disease, sugar and sugar products have been implicated in a wide range of ailments and disorders.

Sugar can cause bone and tooth loss.

According to Dr. Marshall Ringsdorf of the department of oral medicine at the University of Alabama, sugar intake increases calcium elimination from the body. For at least two hours after the intake of one to three ounces of sugar, about 6-18 teaspoons, there is also a reduction in blood phosphorus levels.

The primary function of calcium is to build and maintain bones and teeth in cooperation with phosphorus. After sugar intake, available levels of phosphorus are frequently so low that calcium deposition for bone formation becomes virtually impossible.

Although control of salt intake seems to be the most important factor in treating hypertension, of Dr. James C. Hunt, chairman of the Mayo Clinic's department of medicine, suggests that sugar consumption also seems to have a destructive effect on this condition. Dr. Gerald Berenson of the Louisiana State University School of Medicine, also believes sugar consumption enhances the deleterious effect of salt on blood pressure.

Sugar may also have a harmful effect on the emotions. According to Dr. Bruce Halstead, biotoxicologist and consultant for the World Health Organization, too much dietary sugar can create a depressed, hostile, even suicidal personality.

In the view of Dr. Norman Shealy, neurosurgeon and president of the American Holistic Medical Association, sugar is a major cause of stress. Children and adults with too much sugar in the diet tend toward exaggerated aggressive behavior, frustration, irritability and irrationality.

According to Dr. Richard Ferman, a prominent Californian psychiatrist, at least 43 million Americans are affected by the harmful effects of excess dietary sugar. These people may overreact to situations with their spouses and children, and jeopardize their jobs.

The message is clear: sugar is harmful to many of the body's organ systems as well as our mental and emotional well-being. It must be eliminated from our diet.

CAFFEINE

Stimultants may provide us with spurts of energy but they do not let us know when to rest. (EXECUTIVE FITNESS NEWSLETTER).

Caffeine is a typical stimulant. The amount of caffeine in one to two cups of coffee is sufficient to:

1) Excite all areas of the brain.

2) Dilate the arteries around the heart and the blood vessels around the lungs.

3) Increase the heartbeat and the heart's pumping force.

4) Stimulate stomach acid production.

5) Accelerate kidney activity.

6) Enhance the capacity of skeletal muscles to contract (tighten).

Caffeine provokes the body's internal organs to perform at unhealthy high speeds without furnishing any form of acceptable nourishment at the same time.

The intake of caffeine also triggers a vicious circle. As the initial effects of the caffeine wear off, the usual tendency is to reach for another cup of coffee or another bottle of soda pop. Among the side effects of caffeine intake are sleeping difficulties and thiamine deficiency.

Caffeine sharpens the senses but more often than not we don't know how to utilize our almost painfully-heightened alertness. Irritability, nervousness and muscle twitching are the frequent accompaniments of this alertness.

According to John F. Greden M.D. (AMERICAN JOURNAL OF PSYCHIATRY) excessive caffeine intake may produce symptoms closely resembling those of anxiety neurosis.

CAFFEINE AND RESTLESS LEGS SYNDROME

According to researchers at the Better Sleep Council (NATURAL HEALTH BULLETIN), caffeine may also be responsible for the restless legs syndrome, which afflicts at least one million Americans and is often coupled with insomnia.

Dr. Elmer G. Lutz, chairman of the Department of Neuropsychiatry at St. Mary's Hospital in Passaic, New Jersey, notes that people who begin using or increasing their intake of caffeine in coffee, tea or cola, experience the onset of restless legs syndrome. The primary symptoms include a disagreeable creeping feeling in the lower legs between the ankles and knees, and restlessness in the arms, shoulders and chest muscles. These symptoms occur only when lying down, in the evening or early night.

In mild cases, these symptoms are of brief duration. In moderately serious cases, restless legs syndrome may endure for several hours.

DIET DRINKS

Diet drinks high in caffeine, also have a high chlorine and fluoride content. When either, especially fluoride, is present in excess it can take the place of iodine in the thyroid gland

and create low thyroid levels in the body. A low thyroid level results in feelings of sluggishness. Also, the body's ability to burn up calories is significantly reduced. Efforts to lose weight will then be obstructed.

MARGARINE

After testing the effects of margarine on animals, Fred Rummerow, Ph.D., professor of food science and nutrition at the University of Illinois, has concluded that margarine may cause more hardening of the arteries than butter. Dr. Kummerow considers the dangerous factor in margarine to be trans acid, a fatty acid produced in margarine manufacture.

In the studies in which Dr. Kummerow participated, pigs were fed margarine containing various levels of trans acid. Higher levels of serum cholesterol were discovered in the pigs fed margarine with correspondingly high levels of trans acid. Increased blood cholesterol is linked to atherosclerosis, characterized by fat deposits in large and medium-sized arteries. Serious atherosclerosis may lead to strokes and myocardial infarction or heart attack. Death of heart muscle is due to an inadequate blood supply from the arteries that directly supply, the heart tissue.

Dr. Kummerow has also stated that re-examination of a study of humans, supervised by the National Institutes of Health, demonstrates an increase in serum cholesterol with margarine intake.

ALUMINUM

Avoid aluminum, a mineral found in pans, toiletries, deodorants and certain medications, such as antacids, eye and ear preparations. The concentrations in our environment are wide and varied.

Clinical experiments in Columbus, Ohio, piloted by neuropathologist, Leopold Liss (MEDICAL WORLD NEWS), may be able to confirm the theory that the accumulation of aluminum in the brain causes Alzheimer's disease, a form of insanity which occurs in people over 50.

Large amounts of aluminum have been found in the brains of victims with this form of dementia (madness). A similar brain deterioration has also been produced experimentally in animals receiving this metal.

MILK AND ITS PERILS

Alexander Schauss, director of Biosocial Research in Tacoma, Washington (ORGANIC CONSUMER REPORT) believes that excess intake of milk by children and young adults can end in delinquency.

Schauss contends that children who break the law consistently drink significantly greater amounts of milk than their law-abiding counterparts. Some of these youthful offenders have as many as 14 regular-sized glasses of milk each day.

Investigators at Biosocial Research conducted a study in which a number of chronic offenders were taken completely off milk and dairy products. Within five to six days they had all improved.

In the view of Dr. Kurt Oster, emeritus chief of cardiology at Park City Hospital in Bridgeport, Connecticut (MEDICAL TRIBUNE), homogenized milk is a primary culprit in the development of atherosclerosis or hardening of the arteries. The homogenizing process releases an enzyme which causes the injury.

Skimmed milk may be a good substitute for homogenized milk.

The clinical observations of William A. Ellis, D.O. of Arlington, Texas, (NATIONAL HEALTH FEDERATION BULLETIN) indicate that adults who consume milk products do not absorb nutrients as well as those who avoid milk.

According to Dr. Ellis, milk may be responsible for disorders such as arthritis, asthma, anemia, diarrhea, allergies, migraine headaches, constipation, chronic fatigue, muscle cramps, and obesity, in addition to heart disease.

Resistance to substances which cause allergies, called allergens, is weakened by milk, in Dr. Ellis's view, because few adults can properly break down the protein in cow's milk for use by body cells.

If milk is part of your diet, you are better off with raw, as opposed to pasteurized, milk.

The pasteurization process reduces the B-complex vitamin content of milk by 25 percent and also reduces the content of such minerals as iron. In addition, pasteurization destroys vital enzymes and the antibodies in milk which protect against bacteria.

Chapter XII

Breaking The Smoking Habit: The Case Against Nicotine And Other Poisons

O
n January 11, 1964, the first Surgeon General's report on smoking and health was published.

The report was the first data of irreproachable scientific standing to pinpoint a correlation between smoking, ill-health, and fatal disease.

The tobacco companies spend about 1.8 billion dollars per year globally to advertise cigarettes and smoking. People are thereby "hypnotized" into continuing to smoke.

However, as a result of education programs and persuasive research, more than 30 million Americans have stopped smoking, and the number of cigarettes consumed per capita in America has dropped from 4,345 in 1963 to 3,965 in 1978.

Clearly, dissemination of information by public health agencies, volunteer groups and the media concerning the lethal risks of smoking plays an important role in dissuading people from this addiction.

PINPOINTING THE DANGERS TO THE BODY:
EFFECT ON HEART AND BLOOD VESSELS

Smoking is the major preventable cause of death in America.

Smoking is not merely a personal problem. It has assumed the proportions of a social conflict with repercussions on the economy and on industry.

Smoking is responsible for an annual outlay of five to eight billion dollars in health care expenses. An estimated twelve to eighteen dollars a year are lost in productivity, wages and sick-leave.

With habitual smokers, a decrease in blood circulation to fingers and toes, greater exertion and oxygen consumption by the heart muscles and, a rise in blood pressure and irregular heart rhythms have all been observed, according to the Surgeon General's reports of 1971 and 1975.

These easily-observable effects on the heart and blood vessels produce cumulative long-term effects.

These long-term effects include heart attacks and strokes.

A 1979 report by Dr. Michael Criqui and his colleagues at the University of California School of Medicine in San Diego, indicates smokers have lower levels of HDL, the "good" blood fat, than non-smokers.

A study by John A. Morrison, Ph.D., of the Cincinnati Lipid Research Clinic, revealed immediate, harmful changes in the blood fats of teenage smokers also occur.

CIGARETTE SMOKING AND
CLOGGING OF THE ARTERIES

Cigarette smoking can contribute to clogging of the arteries.

A study by Auerbach, Carter, Garfinkel and Hammond as reported in the journal CHEST (1976), has shown that advanced cases of atherosclerosis, fat deposition in the coronary arteries, were 4.4 times more prevalent in people who had smoked at least 2 packs of cigarettes per day before their deaths than among non-smokers.

Nicotine increases the heart's need for oxygen without increasing the available supply of oxygen.

Nicotine is believed to enhance the sticking together of the platelets of the blood, which are responsible for blood-clotting. Nicotine also seems to obstruct large and small blood vessels, and renders the heart more susceptible to abnormal rhythms called cardiac arrhythmias.

Scientists theorize that people on the margin of cardiac insufficiency can be pushed over that thin line into a heart attack by the effects of nicotine.

In the famous Framingham study, 5209 people have been followed since 1948 in order to correlate lifestyles with the incidence of heart disease. The Framingham researchers have found that in the 50 to 60 age range, smokers are three times more susceptible to heart attacks than non-smokers. In the 60 to 70 range, the incidence is even greater.

SMOKING AND PERIPHERAL VASCULAR DISEASE

Atherosclerotic peripheral vascular disease involves the constriction or obstruction of the arteries of the leg. Arteries in the area of the collar bone, abdomen and kidneys may also be affected by this condition.

The effects of atherosclerotic fat deposition in the leg arteries resemble those in the arteries of the heart. Blood clots that form in the lower leg and foot can cause chronic circulatory problems. These problems may be exacerbated by an immediate need for more blood in any of these areas, for example during exercise.

Research studies have shown a strong connection between peripheral vascular disease and cigarette smoking. A study by N.S. Weiss in THE AMERICAN JOURNAL OF EPIDEMIOLOGY discovered that 70 percent of non-diabetic peripheral vascular disease can be linked to smoking.

Cigarette smoke contains the gas, carbon monoxide (CO). The serious effect of CO on leg cramping is now widely recognized.

SMOKING AND RESPIRATORY DISEASE

The 1964 Surgeon General's Report concluded definitively that cigarette smoking caused lung cancer in men. The less extensive data for women available at that time suggested the same conclusion. The 1964 report also stated that the risk of developing lung cancer increases with the duration of smoking and the quantity of cigarettes smoked daily. Conversely, lung cancer is decreased by giving up smoking completely.

Three subsequent reports by the Public Health Service have confirmed these initial conclusions. The studies cited in these reports demonstrate that the mortality rate from lung cancer among cigarette smokers is approximately ten times greater than that of non-smokers. Cancer of the larynx, oral cavity and esophagus, as well as bronchitis and emphysema, occur more frequently among smokers than among non-smokers.

A study by Dr. Takeshi Hirayama, chief of the National Cancer Center Research Institute in Tokyo, Japan, (MEDICAL WORLD NEWS, February 16, 1981) has shown that non-smoking wifes of middle-aged men who smoked at least 20 cigarettes per day ran a risk of lung cancer death 4.6 times that of women married to non-smokers.

OTHER RESPIRATORY DISEASES AND SYMPTOMS

Adult smokers suffer from respiratory ailments and problems more often than non-smokers. Symptoms, such as hacking coughs, increase in incidence in direct proportion to the increased intake of nicotine.

Not only do smokers have a greater susceptibility to infections of the respiratory tract, but they are also more prone to respiratory complications after surgery.

A study by R.H. Waldman published in the BULLETIN OF THE WORLD HEALTH ORGANIZATION (1969) indicates that people who smoked at least 10 cigarettes per day had an increased susceptibility to flu-like ailments.

Medical research studies indicate that nicotine impedes the production of two kinds of white blood cells. One kind of white blood cell, battles bacteria through the synthesis of substances called antibodies which either inactivate or destroy bacteria. The other kind of white blood cell, produced in the thymus gland fights off cancer and viruses.

BRONCHITIS AND EMPHYSEMA

The frequency of chronic obstructive pulmonary (lung) diseases (COPD) such as chronic bronchitis and emphysema could be sharply reduced if cigarette smoking stopped before age 35.

C.M. Fletcher, R. Peto and C. Tinker ("The natural history of chronic bronchitis and emphysema: An eight year study of early chronic obstructive lung disease in working men in London," OXFORD UNIVERSITY PRESS, 1976), have observed a rapid decrease in lung function as the number of smoking years increases. However, when smoking stopped this sharp decrease in lung function also stopped.

Bronchitis is an affliction of lung tissue known as the bronchi. In bronchitis, there is an overproduction of mucus through extensive exposure to substances that irritate the bronchial passages.

In emphysema, the alveoli are destroyed resulting in the retention of air during the exhalation (breathing out) stage of breathing. When pulmonary emphysema is severe, the airways may totally collapse and prevent the flow of air out of the body.

Bronchitis and emphysema frequently appear in the same person. For this reason it is often difficult to differentiate between these two conditions.

Chronic obstructive pulmonary disease is a major health problem. According to Ruth Winter (THE SCIENTIFIC CASE AGAINST SMOKING, Crown Publishers Inc., New York), it is second only to coronary artery disease as the cause of disabilities compensated by Social Security.

SMOKING AND THE DIGESTIVE SYSTEM

For more than fifty years, evidence has been accumulating in the medical literature of a connection between cigarette smoking and ulcers.

A study by R. Doll, F.A. Johes and F. Pygott, published in the highly respected British journal LANCET (March 29, 1958), investigated the effect of smoking on the development of stomach and intestinal ulcers.

Doll and his colleagues found that 75 percent of those who stopped smoking experienced significant healing of their ulcers compared to only 58 percent of those who went on smoking during the course of the study.

EFFECT OF SMOKING ON ULCERS

According to Dr. David Grimes and Dr. John Goddard of Manchester England (MEDICAL TRIBUNE, 1979), smoking causes accelerated emptying of the stomach after a meal resulting in a more rapid acidification of the intestine. This is significant not only for the development of ulcers but also for the delayed healing of ulcers already present.

DIGESTIVE SYSTEM CANCERS RELATED TO SMOKING

Stomach cancer is twice as prevalent in smokers as in non-smokers. The incidence of cancers of the colon, the lower part of the large intestine, is also greater among smokers.

The digestive process begins in the mouth. Five to ten percent of all cancers develop in this area.

According to Arden G. Christen, D.D.S., M.S.D., author of SMOKING AND YOUR MOUTH: A dentist's view of what smoking may do to the oral cavity. (NARCOTICS EDUCATION, Washington D.C.), approximately 15,000 new cases of cancer of the mouth and throat region are diagnosed every year in the United States. About 90 percent of people afflicted with such cancers use some form of tobacco. The risk of death from oral cancer is four times more likely for smokers than for non-smokers.

The by-products of tobacco also contribute significantly to the formation of heavy deposits around the teeth and to gum disease. A brown or black hair-like coating may be found on the tongue of a smoker. This furlike layer is composed of abnormally thickened and extended projections of the tongue, which tobacco prevents from being shed.

By abstaining from tobacco and tobacco products, these conditions can all be avoided.

BLADDER CANCER

A strong correlation has been established between cigarettes and bladder cancer in both sexes. The risk of bladder cancer increases proportionately with the number of cigarettes smoked daily. In the view of E.L. Wynder and R. Goldsmith (CANCER, 1977), 40 percent of bladder cancer in males and 31 percent of bladder cancer in females can be traced to cigarettes. Workers in the dyestuffs, subber, leather, paint and petroleum industries have an enhanced susceptibility to bladder cancer and this susceptibility is further increased by smoking.

EFFECT OF SMOKING ON NUTRIENTS

According to Dr. W.J. McCormick (ARCHIVES OF PEDIATRICS, October, 1954), smoking enhances our susceptibility to cancer is several ways. For one thing, exposure to the tars in tobacco build-up in the lungs causes a vitamin C deficiency in that area.

What is the connection between vitamin C deficiency and cancer? Nobel laureate Linus Pauling has been experimenting with vitamin C as an anti-carcinogen. William F. Benedict and Peter A. Jones of Children's Hospital in Los Angeles have reported (MEDICAL TRIBUNE) that ascorbic acid, a form of vitamin C, can prevent or reverse the cell changes which usually occur when animal tissue is exposed to cancer-causing agents.

Dr. McCormick's statements regarding the vitamin C-depleting effects of smoking have been confirmed by three scientists whose work was published in the LANCET (March 9, 1963). These scientists compared the blood levels of vitamin C in smoking subjects with blood levels of non-smokers and found that blood levels of vitamin C were significantly lower in smokers.

According to Carl Pfeiffer, M.D., Ph.D. (MENTAL AND ELEMENTAL NUTRIENTS, Keats Publishing Company, 1975), smoking also depletes our supply of thiamine, vitamin B_1. Thiamine is important in the breakdown of carbohydrates for use by the body's cells and also assists in digestion and elimination by maintaining good muscle tone in the digestive tract. Thiamine is essential for a good appetite, healthy growth, and normal functioning of the nervous system.

Further evidence has appeared that a specific eye condition may be cuased by smoking. This condition is amblyopia, or dim vision. Researchers have observed that tobacco-related amblyopia responds to a form of vitamin B_{12}. However, smoking hinders the effectiveness of this form of vitamin B_{12} by lowering both tissue and blood levels.

SIDESTREAM SMOKE:
MORE DANGEROUS THAN MAINSTREAM

Smoking is the main cause of indoor pollution. In many respects, sidestream smoke — the smoke that drifts into the nose, lungs, eyes and blood of non-smokers exposed to the tar and nicotine of smokers — is more poisonous than the smoke inhaled by the smoker, known as mainstream smoke.

Sidestream smoke has 2½ times as much carbon monoxide as mainstream smoke and 73 times as much ammonia. Carbon monoxide blocks absorption of oxygen by blood cells.

Recent studies show that:

1) Sidestream smoke has a harmful effect on small children. Children of smoking parents have more respiratory ailments than children of non-smokers. A study appearing in the American Review of Respiratory Diseases has pinpointed a relation between loss of lung function in children ages six to thirteen and smoking parents.

2) People with heart disease can be gravely affected by even relatively small quantities of carbon monoxide from cigarette smoke.

3) Allergy to tobacco and tobacco smoke exists. Symptoms from this allergy include breathing problems, vomiting, burning eyes, and severe headaches.

4) The smoke that comes off a cigarette is unfiltered smoke and may contain three times as much tar as the smoke that goes through it. This smoke may contain concentrations of cancer-causing agents that are TEN TIMES GREATER than those of smoke that has gone through the cigarette.

5) Chronic exposure to tobacco smoke of other people can produce lung impairment equal to that produced in smokers of one to ten cigarettes per day!

HELPING PEOPLE WHO MUST STOP SMOKING

Many people who are able to stop smoking eliminate

cigarettes gradually. However, as pointed out by Carol June Hooker, R.N., B.S., former Staff Nurse, Hinsdale Sanitorium and Hospital in Hinsdale, Illinois (NURSING Magazine), some people must stop smoking immediately for medical or other reasons.

These people such as a 2-pack-a-day smoker or a pregnant woman at risk for miscarriage, generally have much greater motivation to stop than those smokers who intend to quit "sometime" in the distant future.

The person who must stop smoking immediately should be reminded several times a day, either by a family member, friend or medical professional, of his or her decision to achieve better health, feel better, be more calm, etc. The ability to stop smoking will grow stronger with each repetition of a positive reason never a negative one.

Plentiful amounts of fresh fruits and fluids, such as four to six ounces of freshly squeezed orange juice or bottled or distilled water every waking hour during the first 3 days of not smoking, help eliminate the habitual smoker's high concentrations of nicotine from the body. Decreasing concentrations of nicotine only stimulates a craving for more, so it is best that nicotine be expelled as quickly and thoroughly as possible.

Taking slow deep breaths when a craving to smoke arises relaxes the body long enough to sustain the decision not to smoke. In addition, this breathing technique teaches how to supply body and brain with sufficient oxygen.

Several slow deep breaths should be taken with the mouth wide open. Bending from the waist aids in exhaling, preferably with lips pursed.

Coffee, tea and colas contain caffeine which stimulates the urge to smoke and should be avoided.

Vinegar, mustard and pepper may also provoke the urge to smoke in some cases.

B VITAMINS AND EXERCISE

Extra rest and supplemental B vitamins, especially thiamine, can assist in preventing the nervousness and irritability that may result from strenuous efforts to stop smoking.

Brewer's yeast can be a good source of the B vitamins.

Exercise, such as brisk walking, can also help prevent irritability and depression and improve blood circulation.

Chain smokers often need to keep their hands occupied while quitting. Pipe-cleaner figures, carrot sticks and apple wedges are all useful, and in the last two cases, nutritious, distractions for restless fingers.

Chewing a piece of raw ginger root can help satisfy the need for a bitter taste.

The person who is giving up smoking may be irritable and anxious, and complain of headaches, dizziness, diminished attention span, loss of appetite, drowsiness, lethargy, muscle cramps and increased sweating.

Spiritual and emotional support is of great value during the quitting period.

Chapter XIII

Cytotoxic Testing For Food Allergy

A growing number of physicians in the United States, Canada and Britain are convinced that food allergies contribute to a wide variety of illnesses and degenerative diseases such as arthritis, alcoholism, high blood presure, and schizophrenia.

Both physical and emotional problems may develop from the body's intolerance to some of the foods we consume.

Over twelve years ago, Dr. Marshall Mandell, presently director of the Alan Mandell Center for Bio-Ecologic Diseases, noted that certain food extracts could produce a vast array of bodywide allergic symptoms in patients with respiratory allergies. These symptoms included joint and muscle pain, depression, headache, fatigue, confusion, and bowel and bladder problems.

From his experience with patients, Dr. Donald J. Carrow has found that food allergies may produce learning disorders, overweight, compulsive eating patterns, and nervousness, and that an appropriate change in diet can cure migraine headaches, eczema, ichthisis (fish skin disease) abnormal heart thythms (cardiac arrhythmias), and aggressive behavior.

Dr. R.O. Brennan, founder of the International Academy of Preventive Medicine and author of several books on nutrition, believes that most people have allergies as a result of poor diet and careless eating habits.

RESISTANCE TO THE CONCEPTS OF FOOD ALLERGY AND CYTOXIC TESTING

All too often the simplest and most effective concepts in health and medicine encounter a great deal of resistance before they are accepted. Such has been the case with both food allergy and cytotoxic testing for food allergy.

Most physicians admit that people can be allergic to inhaled pollen or certain drugs. Too many, however, do not accept the concept that allergic reactions may result from the consumption of specific foods and chemicals, or that disturbances in the muscles, nerves, gastrointestinal tract, inner ear and sex organs, as well as the more familiar nose, throat, lung and skin symptoms, may make up part of these allergic reactions.

These physicians are similarly ignorant regarding the concept of cytotoxic testing for food allergy. They are quick to defend the traditional methods for detecting food allergy such as the prick or scratch test instead.

The prick method is inadequate for detecting food allergy.

Among the rapidly expanding number of physicians who firmly support the use of cytotoxic food testing for food allergy are Dr. John H. Boyle, Jr., M.D., Assistant Professor of otorhinolaryngology at Wright State University and Dr. Brennan. Otorhinolaryngology is the medical specialty which deals with ear, nose and larynx-related disorders.

UNDERSTANDING THE CYTOTOXIC APPROACH

The word "cytotoxic" is derived from the Greek and means "having a poisonous effect on body cells." The name is related to the fact that certain foods and chemicals can have a harmful effect on body cells." The name is related to the fact that certain foods and chemicals can have a harmful effect on specific white blood cells known as neutrophils. Upon contact with the offending food, these cells may either change their structure or be completely destroyed.

In cytotoxic testing, first devised by Arthur P. Black, M.D., "A New Diagnostic Method in Allergic Disease", a blood sample is obtained from the person being tested. This form of allergy testing is therefore an **in vitro,** or outside the body, mode of testing. It does not require further patient involvement after the blood sample has been drawn.

White cells are extracted from the blood sample and placed on a microscopic slide that contains the food to be tested. A video camera reveals whether the blood cells' reaction to the food is slight, moderate or severe, after a 45-minute incubation period.

A LARGE NUMBER OF POSSIBLY OFFENDING SUBSTANCES MAY BE TESTED THROUGH CYTOTOXIC TESTING

In the view of Jeffrey Zavik, a technician skilled in cytotoxic testing and an assistant to Dr. Brennan, one dramatic advantage of cytotoxic testing is that so many substances can be screened in a short period of time.

Reactions to 144 substances can be measured in one day as compared to the three or four skin tests performed during one visit to the doctor's office.

THE ROTARY DIET

About 15% of foods consistently produce allergies. These foods must be permanently avoided. The remaining 85% will cause allergies only if they are consumed too often. Such allergies are known as cyclic allergies.

Sensitivity reactions to most foods may be eliminated with a rotary diversified diet. On such a diet, a food capable of causing an allergic reaction is eaten only at 4-6 day intervals and avoided in-between.

SCIENTIFIC STUDY OF THE CYTOTOXIC FOOD TEST

John H. Boyles, Jr., M.D. ("The Validity of Using the Cytotoxic Food Test in Clinical Allergy", INSIGHT PUBLISHING COMPANY, 1977) first used the cytotoxic food test in 1972.

Dietary lists and instructions were furnished to patients and follow-up was provided by a competent technician.

A questionnaire was sent to 239 patients with food allergies to determine the success of the cytotoxic therapy program.

Among these patients, nasal congestion, headaches, nasal discharge, and recurring inflammation of the sinuses were the four most prevalent ear, nose and throat symptoms of food allergy. Watery eyes, dizziness, sore throat, fullness in the head, ringing in the ears, a cough, breathing problems, loss of hearing, recurrent ear infections, gagging, itching ear and ear drainage were the other common ear, nose and throat symptoms. For each symptom, more than 50% of patients experienced relief through proper diet.

OTHER FOOD ALLERGY SYMPTOMS RELIEVED

As revealed by the questionnaire, the most common food allergy symptoms relieved by crtotoxic therapy and proper diet were fatigue, bloating after meals, mental depression, abdominal pain, eye trouble, diarrhea, and skin rash.

Many patients suffering from these symptoms indicated they experienced relief for the first time in many years and after a vast array of alternative treatments had proved futile.

SMOKING AND ALCOHOL

The cure rate for food allergy was 50% lower among smokers that among people who had never smoked or had stopped smoking. Smoking is probably the most dangerous habit any allergic patient can have.

Dr. Boyle also found that food allergic patients must not use alcohol frequently and should be restricted to those beverages distilled from a food to which they are not allergic. Most alcoholic beverages contain yeast, malt, barley, hops, corn, rye and sugar.

Chapter XIV

Exercise: Another Vital Component Of The Holistic Balanced Treatment

*E*xercise serves many functions. It can build muscle tone and strength, reduce tension, aid in weight loss, and improve overall physiological condition, especially the heart's capacity to furnish oxygen to body tissues.

Exercise helps maintain physical, emotional and mental well-being.

As pointed out by Jane Brody, science editor for THE NEW YORK TIMES, particular kinds of exercise may fulfill some needs but not others.

THE DIFFERENT KINGS OF EXERCISE: ISOMETRIC, ISOTONIC, AEROBIC

There are two fundamental kinds of strength-building exercises: isometric exercise and isotonic exercise. Isometric exercise contracts individual muscles undergoing exercise without movement of that body part.

Isotonic exercise involves movement such as lifting weights.

Neither isometric or isotonic exercise is designed to improve the efficiency of the heart and lungs. Sustained body movement such as walking, bicycling, swimming and running is needed. These activities belong in the group of aerobic, or air-dependent, exercise.

The fit person breathes more efficiently than the unfit person during exertion. The fit person's resting heartbeat is lower and more stable. With exercise, less lactic acid, a substance which induces fatigue, is produced. Aerobic exercise can also lower blood pressure, and blood triglyceride levels.

THE PARTICULAR BENEFITS OF WALKING

Walking is the most popular form of adult exercise in the United States, according to a national fitness study released in 1979 entitled "Fitness in America".

When we walk every moving part of our body moves naturally, as nature intended.

Muscles stretch and turn with each step, stimulating circulation and helping the heart to pump blood.

Brisk walking improves the pumping of oxygen-laden blood to the brain. As larger quantities of fresh oxygen are delivered to brain cells, mental alertness is strengthened.

Walking is now accepted as effective treatment for the injured heart. At the Longevity Center in Santa Monica, California, treatment consists of a low-fat diet and mandatory walking. Brisk walking, which burns 300 calories per hour, can assist in losing weight and reducing hip bulge.

Walking can function either as a tranquillizer or stimulant, reducing tension, anger, and other negative emotions, as well as the pressure of everyday problems.

A three-day symposium on Exercise in Aging held at the National Institute of Health in Bethesda, Maryland, concluded that walking is the safest and most effective form of exercise.

Walk with your feet parallel and pointing forward, your abdomen flat, your back straight and your head erect. Make sure your whole foot touches the ground as you walk — heal first, then toes — at a pace that makes your heart beat faster and induces deeper breathing.

HOW TO IMPROVE POSTURE

A healthy, youthful and attractive appearance depends on a sound diet, positive emotional outlook, sufficient rest and good posture.

At any age, the primary obstacle to good posture is the downward pulling forces of gravity.

Good posture results from good balance, with the weight evenly distributed from heels to the balls of the feet and toes.

The arches of your feet should be relaxed and raised slightly on the inside with ankles at the same horizontal level, as knees, hips, shoulders, ears and eyes.

Your arms should hang in a relaxed manner with hands and fingertips level. Your head should be evenly positioned between the shoulders according to both side and front views.

A technique called "imaging" used in ballet, yoga and sports medicine can be useful. Try to focus on an image of perfect posture which you would like to imitate.

Imagine balloons filled with helium attached to the parts of your body you wish to control or move. Link these balloons to your favorite colors. Ultimately, each time you see that color you will imagine a successful lift.

EXERCISE WILL NOT INCREASE YOUR APPETITE

A study by U.S. and British nutrition researchers of six overweight women has revealed that exercise does not increase appetite.

Women participating in the study, conducted by Columbia University nutritionist Dr. Rosy Woo, performed very little exercise over a 19 day period, followed by light exercise over a second 19 day period, and heavy exercise during a final 19 day period. During each of the three periods, the women were permitted to eat as much as they wished.

Calorie intake changed only slightly no matter how strenuously the participants in the study exercised. At the study's termination, the women were burning about 500 calories more a day than they had when not exercising.

EXERCISE AND ARTHRITIS

For the person with arthritis, regular exercise and activity once symptoms begin to disappear can prevent crippling deformity, help restore joint movement, and stimulate healing of arthritis-injured tissue. As a result of exercise, heart, blood vessels, muscles, nerves and glands will function more efficiently.

Exercises should be performed slowly and frequently. A leisurely approach protects against unnecessary strain and injury and allows for maximum psychological and spiritual benefit. Exercise should never be permitted to cause discomfort, nor should activity be an occasion for frantic competitiveness — especially against oneself.

As symptoms begin to subside, physicians skilled in administering the Holistic Balanced Treatment recommend deep breathing, from the abdomen as opposed to the chest, moderate stretching, swimming, use of a rocking chair to stimulate mild rhythmic muscular contraction and improve circulation of the blood, and everyday walking about the house.

This is a prelude to more complex and demanding straightening and extending exercises, advisable only when pain, tenderness, stiffnes and soreness have been fairly well eliminated.

EXERCISING: THE BEST TIMES AND PLACES

The best times to exercise are before breakfast, late afternoon, and at least one and a half hours after dinner. The space reserved for exercise should be congenial — a kind of sanctuary free from intrusive stimuli.

When exercising requires you to lie on your back, you should make sure the space set aside for this purpose contains a sufficiently wide flat surface. This surface should be covered with a comfortable mat or blanket for the duration of exercise. All objects and clothing that hinder freedom of movement should be removed.

EXERCISES FOR THE PERSON WITH ARTHRITIS

Listed below are a series of exercises which have been effectively utilized by patients receiving the Holistic Balanced Treatment. At first, most patients perform these exercises three times a day. The number of repetitions per day may be increased gradually as symptoms are eliminated.

Patients find that the persistence of pain and discomfort several hours after the completion of the exercises is a sign that exertion has been excessive. Regular, limited, but slowly increasing periods of exercise are of much greater therapeutic value than long periods of strain and stress resulting in inordinate pain and fatigue.

EXERCISES FOR THE HAND

1. Without lifting the forearm off the surface of a table, crumple a large sheet of newspaper with the fingers. Try to get as much paper into the ball as possible.

2. Tear a paper in half, then into quarters, eights, etc. Strive to create a maximum number of strips.

3. Several commercial clays and therapeutic putties are available commercially. These are all satisfactory. The consistency of Play-Doh, however, allows for finer finger movements.

Flatten the Play-Doh and place the hand, palm down, against it with the fingers placed close together. Try to separate the fingers against the resistance furnished by the Doh. If the exercise proves too difficult at first, a therapist or friend should be recruited to supply resistance against attempts to stretch the fingers apart.

Squeeze the Play-Doh with your fingers.

The Play-Doh can be flattened like a pancake (½" thick) with palms down and joints flexed so that fingertips are in contact with the material. Against the resistance of the Doh, push with all five fingers until the entire hand is flat on the table.

The Play-Doh can be squeezed into a ball. Begin rolling your hand over the Doh, from palm outward to fingertips and back again. In this manner, a long Doh cylinder will be formed. The exercise should be performed with a light touch and good movement in the joints. Locking shoulder and elbow joints and supplying thrust from the trunk defeats the purpose of this exercise.

After rolling the Play-Doh, roll a pencil in the same manner, but only when muscle strength and tone in both hand and forearm are good. This exercise hinges on the interplay of extension (stretching) and flexion (bending) movements in the hand rather than on flatness and rigidity.

4. Writing exercises are helpful in improving strength of hand muscles. Hold a pen or pencil and begin movement at the level of the shoulder. The writing space should be equivalent in height to two lines of type. Movements should begin by producing large connected circles which gradually diminish in size. Movements should be carried out with exaggerated slowness until pure finger writing is achieved.

5. Rest the forearm on a table with the palm of the hand raised upward. The hand should extend beyond the table edge so that it can move up and down freely. With your forearm resting on the table at all times, lift your hand as high as possible and keep it in a fixed position for five seconds. Slowly lower the hand as far as it will go.

6. With the forearm resting on the table top and the palm positioned downward, the hand, once again, freely extended beyond the table edge to allow for unrestrained vertical movement—raise the hand as high as possible holding it tightly in a raised

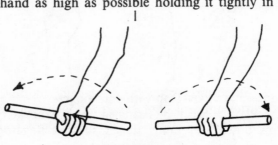

position for a count of five. Then slowly lower it as far as it will go.

This exercise five and six promote improved wrist flexion and extension.

EXERCISES FOR THE FINGERS

1. With the hand placed palm downward on a table and fingers over the edge, allow fingers to bend downward in the direction of the floor. Keeping the palm flat on the table surface, try to bend the fingers at the joints.

2. With the palm placed downward on the table, try to raise the fingers up from the table as high as possible. Hold them in that position for a count of three then lower them to the starting position.

3. With the hand resting palm upward on the table, bring the fingertips in toward the palm as far as possible. Hold them in a stretched position for three seconds then bring them back to the initial position.

4. With the hand open and palm up, place a soft sponge or rolled-up washcloth in the palm and squeeze as tightly as possible. Hold the hand in this tightened position for three seconds, then release.

5. Sprinkle powder on the table surface to reduce friction With the hand resting palm downward on the table, keep the little, ring and middle fingers stationary and move the index finger away from these three toward the thumb as far as possible. Return index finger to the initial position.

6. Open your hand, then clench. The fingers should be spread widely as the hand is opened. Touch each finger to the thumb, planting each firmly against it.

EXERCISES FOR ELBOWS AND SHOULDERS

1. With the palm of the hand on the table and forearm elevated straight up from the table top, try to raise your elbow as high as possible while exerting pressure on the table top with your palm.

2. Stand erect with elbows at your sides and slowly flex your forearms upwards until fingertips touch shoulders.

3. Place your hands behind your head and draw your

elbows back as far as they will go. At the same time try to pull in your chin and draw back your head.

4. Face the wall and place your hands against the wall surface. Keeping your feet in place, push the upper part of your trunk toward the wall, flexing your elbows as you advance. Make your hands touch your shoulders. Return to initial position and repeat the exercise.

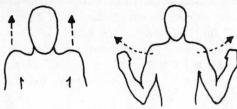

5. Shrug shoulders upward, downward, and then in a circular movement.

6. Adopt a stance halfway between standing erect and stooping. Let your arms dangle. Rock your body back and forth at the hips.

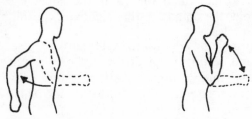

7. Extend your arms sideways with elbows bent so that the upper arms are at right angles to forearms. Try to swing hands and forearms downward and then upward. In this way, the shoulder joints will rotate.

8. Lying face-down on your bed, clasp your hands behind your neck. Raise your head and elbows upward as you keep the rest of your body fixed. Repeat.

EXERCISES FOR KNEES AND HIPS

1. Seated in bed, move your leg outward as far as possible. Keep your knees straight and toes pointed outward.

2. Sitting on a chair, draw each knee up as close as possible to the chest. Lower each knee and extend the corresponding leg outward. If you are seated with your legs dangling over the edge of a chair, friend or therapist may be able to furnish resistance against the leg extension.

3. Lying on your back with legs straight, try to slide your legs apart. Then, try to raise and lower each leg from the same straight position.

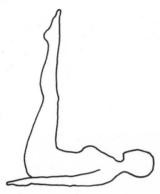

4. Lying on your stomach, lift your leg, bending the knee as much as possible.

5. Hold on the back of a chair. Raise your right leg in front without bending your knee. Slowly move it to the side, then bring it back in a full circle, returning leg to the front. Repeat slowly ten times. Do the same movement with the other leg.

EXERCISES FOR FEET

1. Sitting with soles flat on the floor, first raise your toes, then your heels. Then, turn your soles inward facing each other.

2. Sitting in a chair or on a stool, try to pick up a cloth with your toes. Carry it between your toes to the opposite hand.

3. Push the ball of the foot against a ged rail or fixed bar in a lying flat position. Bend and spread the toes alternately.

4. Bend the foot forward, then backward, in a lying flat position.

GENERAL FUNCTIONAL ACTIVITIES

There are several everyday functions and activities which have exercise value. These include:

1) Washing dishes, especially in warm water. Bending and straightening your fingers is necessary during plate, dishrag and towel manipulation.

2) Kneading dough. This activity is extremely effective in strengthening hand movements. However, wrist pain or severely limited range of motion in the wrist is a definite sign **not** to do this exercise.

3) Beating eggs. Beating eggs with a hand-held rotary egg beater is excellent for developing finger and wrist muscles.

4) Wringing towels. This improves wrist and forearm movements, and strengthens the grip.

THE HEAD-DROP METHOD

The self-relaxing head-drop method is one way of combining psychological self-help with exercise. This holistic approach induces a state of relaxation throughout the body, enabling joints to feel loose and relaxed.

In the head-drop method, the head is elevated and kept elevated for 2 minutes from a position flat on the back. Two deep breaths are taken with the eyes closed to eliminate all tension from the body. Gradually the head is lowered back to its original position and goes limp.

Then imagine that your right arm is stiffening to the point of complete numbness. The "anesthesia" induced in the arm can then be extended to other parts of the body. When accompanied by the suggestion that muscles and joints are becoming easier to move the "anesthesia" will decrease pain and stiffness and enable joints to move more freely.

The person utilizing the head-drop method must avoid the stress of negative emotions such as anxiety, rage, jealousy and depression, and focus on such positive fellings as self-acceptance, forgiveness, and love of self and others. Pleasant thoughts, for example, soothing country scenes, music and direct suggestions that pain is being relieved will help you avoid stress.

Joints will soon begin to feel loose and relaxed through the influence of body on mind and mind on body.

SOME MORE ADVANCED EXERCISES
GEARED TO HOLISTIC WELL-BEING

In addition to the exercises listed above, there is a wide range of additional exercises that can be performed to achieve well-being of mind, body and spirit. These include the following:

STRENGTHENING AND RELAXING
PELVIC AND LOWER BACK MUSCLES

Stand relaxed with your feet apart. With hands on your hips and breathing deeply, move your hips in a wide arc. Use your pelvis muscles to regulate the motion. Without straining, try to move your hips in the widest possible arcs.

GIVING FLEXIBILITY TO SPINE,
NECK AND TORSO MUSCLES

Lie on your stomach with your forehead touching the floor. With your palms touching the floor and elbows raised just a little, raise your head and trunk. The lower half of the body should retain contact with the floor. Inhale deeply as you perform this exercise taking care not to strain excessively. With the upper part of your body raised, wait seven seconds before lowering your body — first trunk, then head.

This exercise, in which the upper part of your body becomes a smooth curve from crown to lower back, renders the deep and surface muscles of the back more supple. The stress-laden abdomen relaxes and blood circulation improves.

RELAXING ABDOMEN AND PELVIS

This exercise can help alleviate such conditions as constipation.

As you lie flat on your back with your arms at your sides, relax and inhale deeply. As you inhale, flex your knee and bring it toward your chest. Without straining lock your hands about your knee in a position not far from the chest.

113

Breathing deeply, wait eight seconds, then release your knee and lower it smoothly to the floor.

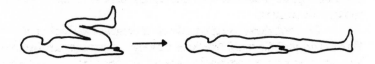

GIVING ELASTICITY TO
SHOULDER AND NECK MUSCLES

Sitting upright in a comfortable armchair, relax and breathe deeply. Elevate your shoulders toward your ears and out in front of your chest in a gentle unstrained manner. After you have gently lowered your shoulders back to the normal position, draw your shoulders behind your chest so that shoulder blades move toward each other. make sure that you do not strain. You can perform these elevating/rotating movements several times.

COMPREHENSIVE MUSCLE AND JOINT RELAXATION

Lying on your back, extend your arms straight out from your body. Bend your knees and draw them toward your chest without straining. Keep the heels of your feet near your buttocks and slightly elevated. Now, turning your lower body to the right, turn your head to the left, without forcing any portion of your body. The key is gentleness. Turn your head and lower body back to their normal position and reverse directions — head to the right, buttocks and legs to the left. You will be enhancing muscle tone in the spine and massaging the abdomen.

EXERCISE AND THE OFFICE WORKER

People who sit for hours each day hunched over paperwork, typewriters, and telephones, frequently develop a slump or slouch which becomes more conspicuous with time. This slouching is a major cause of the familiar hump which becomes so crippling and disfiguring in later years.

According to Dr. Howard F. Hunt, chairman of the physical education department at the University of California at

San Diego, office slump is traceable to a failure to invest the energy needed to "sit and walk tall". As upper body muscles become tighter and shorter, the slump becomes more and more difficult to correct.

Dr. Willibald Nagler, physiotherapist-in-chief at the New York Hospital-Cornell Medical Center, recommends the following set of exercises specially geared to the posture problems of the office worker. They are designed to combat upper-back pain and should be done three or more times a week:

The first three are rapid relaxers to be performed lying on one's back on a bed or exercise mat with a pillow beneath the knees.

1) Breathe in through the nose. Exhale slowly through pursed lips. Repeat five times.

2) Roll your head gently from side to side making no effort to sustain any one position. Repeat ten times.

3) Raise shoulders up toward the ears, then allow them to drop completely. Repeat ten times.

4) Standing, place your palms on your chest. Pull your shoulders down. Bring your elbows to shoulder level and rotate your arms ten times clockwise, then ten times counterclockwise.

5) Lie on your back on a bed or exercise mat. Placing your hands behind your neck, bring your elbows down to the exercise surface and press downward very hard. Hold this pose for five seconds, then relax. Repeat ten times.

6) On a bed or exercise mat, descend on all fours with your back straight and elbows locked. Your hands should point forward with the palms down. Shift position and sit on your haunches keeping your hands in place but palms turned upwards. Hold for five seconds. Repeat ten times.

7) In a sitting position, hold a two-and-a-half pound weight in your right hand. Put the hand over your left hip, keeping your arm as straight as possible. Raise the weight in a straight line from hip to shoulder. Try to reach backwards. Hold for five seconds. Repeat the exercise with the other arm. Perform the exercise five times with each arm.

PREGNANCY AND EXERCISE

According to Debi Armstrong, RN, who leads a class in

deep breathing relaxation and exercise for pregnant mothers in Tampa, Florida, exercise may help alleviate some of the unpleasant side effects of pregnancy, including circulatory problems, edema (tissue swelling) and congestion in the pelvic area. Exercise also helps prepare a woman for the strenous work of labor and delivery and speeds recovery after birth.

Utilizing some stretching and bending, Nurse Armstrong concentrates on those body areas that enlarge during pregnancy, buttocks, abdomen and thighs. Exercises that induce excessive abdominal pressure, such as full sit-ups and double leg lifts, are to be avoided, along with the jolting movements associated with aerobics.

EXERCISING DURING BUSINESS TRAVEL

There are several ways to stay limber and refreshed despite all the inconveniences of air travel.

According to Shelley Liebman, director of The Home Stretch, a fitness organization based in the nation's capital, air travel-related fitness begins with an intelligent approach to luggage.

Try packing two smaller pieces instead of one large piece of luggage. This will insure equal distribution of weight as you carry your bags and will eliminate neck, arm and back strain.

After a lengthy flight as you wait for luggage to be unloaded, stretch arms, neck and back. Always lift luggage with the knees bent.

Wear comfortable footwear made of leather or other natural materials that breathe and shock-absorbent rubber soles for extensive walking in large airports.

EXERCISING ON PLANE

To relieve pressure on your back, keep knees higher than your hips. Walk around as much as possible.

To relieve shoulder tension, rotate your shoulders forward, then backwards. Conclude by lifting your shoulders up to your ears.

To stretch your back, lower your head and raise your knees until they meet. Hold for five seconds, then relax.

To strengthen your arms, place both hands on the seat in front of you with arms extended and push. Hold for five seconds, then release.

To strengthen your abdomen, inhale and pull stomach muscles toward your back. Hold for four seconds, exhale.

EXERCISE AND YOUR ACHING BACK

Common backache is a general condition affecting up to 70 million Americans.

Most of the time the source of the problem is an excessively weak or strong muscle, not necessarily located in the back, which places an abnormal stress on another muscle. After compensating for a certain period of time the muscle will begin to hurt because of strain or fatigue. A chain reaction may develop.

Since the back is a centrally-situated fulcrum for a vast array of body movements, it ultimately feels the effects of the chain reaction.

According to Dr. Hans Kraus, Manhattan-based authority on back pain and author of several books on the subject, 80 percent of lower back pain comes from muscle deficiency. Dr. Kraus emphasizes the role of the abdominal muscles. When they are weak, the back muscles must make an unnatural compensatory effort and begin to hurt.

In the view of Dr. Martin Feldman, a New York neurologist, many back problems originate in the feet. When the feet and ankles are not properly aligned, stress is transmitted unevenly throughout the body causing misalignment of the spine and back pain.

Dr. Richard Bachrach, also of New York, considers the recognition of emotional stress and psychological factors the most significant recent breakthrough in back pain treatment.

EXERCISES FOR BACK PAIN

Dr. William F. Donaldson, Jr., medical director of Children's Hospital in Pittsburgh and former president of the Academy of Orthopedic Surgeons, believes that keeping one's weight down, maintaining good posture and avoiding too much sitting are crucial in eliminating or reducing back pain.

Dr. Donaldson also recommends the following 5 exercises for back pain:

1) Lying on your back, suck in your stomach muscles as tightly as you can. Hold them for a count of five.

2) Lying on your back, lift your head off the ground until you can see your feet.

3) Lying on your back with your arms at your side and your knees bent, lift your head and back off the floor as far as you can without putting unnecessary strain on your lower back.

4) Lying on your back with your arms at your sides, and your knees bent, lift your entire trunk and upper part of your body until your tead touches your knees.

5) Lying on your back with legs flat on the floor, raise one knee to chest, pressing it against the chest using both arms. Then resume the initial position. Repeat this exercise with the other knee. Then, attempt it with both knees simultaneously.

BACK PAIN THERAPY WITH A SLANT BOARD

Dr. Ernest Johnson, professor and chairman of the physical medicine department at Ohio State University, finds sit-ups done on a slant board, available at discount chain stores, can dramatically alleviate back pain by strengthening stomach muscles. These muscles are the sole support for the five lower lumbar vertebrae (spinal bones) implicated in lower back pain.

The sit-ups should be done with the knees bent so that the backs of the heels touch the buttocks. Dr. Johnson advises starting slowly and progressing gradually to 20 sit-ups per day.

The height of the slant board should be increased regularly by 4 inches until 20 sit-ups are being performed comfortably at 16 inches.

A POSTURE GEARED TO REDUCING BACK PAIN

Two orthopedic surgeons, Dr. Hamilton Hall, assistant professor of surgery at the University of Toronto, and Dr. Vert Mooney of the University of Texas, recommend a "drinking man's pub posture" — with one foot raised off the floor on a bar rail — to relieve back pain and induce relaxation.

Raising one foot — on a bar rail or suitable substitutes such as a box, low table, footstool, low drawer or thick telephone directory — alters the curve of the back thereby relieving some of the extra stress on the lower back.

According to the surgeons, the person maintaining this stance should stand in the most comfortable position and keep alternating the foot that is elevated.

PROPER LIFTING TO AVOID IMPAIRMENT OF THE BACK

As pointed out by Bernice Doyle Owen, R.N., M.S.N. ("How to Avoid that Aching Back", AMERICAN JOURNAL OF NURSING), more than 50 percent of job-related back injuries can be traced directly to incorrect bending and lifting methods.

You can reduce the risk of such injury by applying the following principles to lifting:

a) Keep the load close to your body.

b) Plant your body so that as many muscle groups as possible can work together in harmony and balance. For example, if you are going to lift a load of sheets from a low shelf to a waist-high receptacle, begin with the back and knees bent. Use the muscles in your arms and shoulders to pull the lumbar, abdominal and thigh muscles for the crucial upward lift. If you are lifting sheets from a high shelf to a higher one, keep your back straight and let the arm and shoulder muscles join with those of the thigh, abdomen and lumbar region for the lift.

The term **lumbar** refers to the part of the back and sides between the ribs and pelvis. The lumbar muscle group includes muscles that surround the bones in the lumbar, or lower back, region of the spine and connect with the pelvis and back ribs.

c) Consider an object excessively heavy if it is 35 percent of your body weight. If you plan to carry an object weighting more than ten pounds, make sure the object has handles located above its approximate dead center. If you plan to carry bulky objects, make sure they weigh no more than twenty pounds.

A new lifting technique proposed by safety experts makes the following additional recommendations:

1. When lifting, keep the feet about a shoulder's width apart for good leverage.

2. The back should be in a bent position and the knees partially bent. When you lift, the arm and shoulder muscles pull; the lumbar and abdominal muscles are contracted for both pull and leverage. The thigh and leg muscles furnish the upward thrust to bring the object to the level of the knees.

3. To lift further, begin to straighten your knees. Keep the back flexed and the lumbar and abdominal muscles tightened.

4. When you lift further, from mid-thigh to waist level, flex your knees for more upward thrust, begin to straighten your back, and bring the object to be lifted closer to the body. At this point, it is the leg and thigh muscles which effect the actual lifting.

5. When lifting is complete, the knees and back are in a less bent but not a straight position.

6. When lowering an object from waist level to the floor, carry out the above steps in reverse order to insure that the body's muscles work in a balanced synchronized fashion and thereby avoid lumbar strain.

7. Back injury can also occur when a twisting movement is performed during lifting. Avoid twisting completely. Instead, try to pivot with your whole body. Since the new lifting technique recommends placing the feet a shoulder width apart, balance can be maintained during whole body pivoting.

8. When an object is too heavy, ask for assistance to make several trips.

9. When working close to the ground, kneel. Never bend over.

10. Before you lift, make sure your path is unobstructed, free of hazards, and that your feet are securely entrenched.

EXERCISES AND EXERCISING
TECHNIQUES: THAT TO AVOID

Flexibility should be the result of gentle, natural strengthening and training of the muscles around joints.

According to Richard H. Dominguez, M.D., instructor of orthopedic surgery at Loyola University Medical Center and author of TOTAL BODY TRAINING, flexibility through unnatural stretching has become an end in itself.

When joints are bent beyond the ability to control them with muscle strength, the risk of tearing the muscles, tendons and ligaments that support the joint is greatly enhanced. In addition, there is a danger of injuring the joint surface by exerting abnormal pressure on it.

A tendon is a cord of tough fibery connective tissue through which muscles are attached to bones. A ligament is a band of tough tissue which usually connects bone to bone or holds an organ in place.

There are several stretch exercises that should be completely eliminated from the exerciser's repertoire. These do not contribute to overall fitness and to the strengthening of the back and may lead to injury in many people.

1) YOGA PLOW: This exercise puts excessive pressure on spinal disks and ligaments and may cause irreversible fiber injury in the base of the spine and in the sciatic nerve. The spinal disks are composed of layers of fibrous connective tissue with small masses of cartilage among the fibers. They are found between vertebrae, or spinal bones.

In addition, the yoga plow causes extreme stress to the blood vessels servicing the brain and upper spinal cord, making the possibility of a stroke frighteningly real.

2) HURDLER'S STRETCH: This exercise stretches the ligaments and muscles of the groin to an excessive degree, and may lead to chronic groin pull. Hurdler's stretch can also injure the cartilage of the knee joint and produce a constant long-term pull on the ligament which helps stabilize the knee.

3) DUCK WALK AND DEEP KNEE-BEND: Waddling in a duck-like manner in a deep-knee position can cause excruciating pain through tears in knee cartilage.

4) TOE TOUCHING: Serious damage to both the posterior longitudinal ligament, one of the primary supporting ligaments of the spine, and the sciatic nerve can happen with this exercise. Contrary to what many exercisers believe, the toe touching exercise, instead of relaxing the back, actually tightens its muscles.

5) BALLET STRETCHES: Ballet stretches can damage

the back of the knee, as well as the ligaments, muscles, joints and discs clustered in the lower back. This exercise also produces sharp pains along the legs as a result of excessive stretching of the sciatic nerve fibers.

6) STIFF LEG RAISE: This exercise also stretches the sciatic nerve far beyond normal bounds.

7) KNEE STRETCH: This patently harmful exercise destabilizes the knees by putting excessive strain on two important knee ligaments.

8) SIT-UPS: In Dr. Dominguez's view, sit-ups, designed to strengthen muscles of the abdomen, actually shorten those muscles after a certain point. In addition, sit-ups produce back strain and abnormal nerve lengthening.

Chapter XV
The Therapeutic Value Of Sex For Arthritis

Sexual activity can be helpful in the treatment of arthritis. A study of 55 people with arthritis conducted at the Sexual Dysfunction Clinic of Chicago's Cook County Hospital revealed a positive effect of sex on arthritis. Twenty-four participants interviewed experienced enhanced general well-being and relief of arthritis pain after sexual activity.

According to Wanda Sadoughi, Ph.D., director of the Chicago clinic, many of the patients, whose ages ranged from the twenties to late sixties, said that they were completely "free of pain for several hours" after engaging in sexual relations.

Dr. Jesse E. Potter, director of the National Institute for Human Relationships in Chicago (MEDICAL WORLD NEWS), believes sex may give four to six hours of relief from the pain of arthritis.

Dr. Potter, who lectures on human sexuality at both the University of Illinois and Northwestern University Medical School, is careful to emphasize that sex as a pain reliever does not necessarily mean sexual intercourse.

Any form of sexual stimulation which triggers the release of the hormone cortisone is good for arthritis pain. The quality of sexual experience also plays a role in determining the extent of relief. For example, sex with someone who induces negative emotions can have a correspondingly negative effect on painful or inflamed joints.

STIMULATING THE ADRENAL

The mechanism by which sex alleviates the pain of arthritis is not completely understood.

In the view of Dr. George E. Ehrlich, professor of medicine at Temple University, in Philadelphia, Pennsylvania, sex probably acts as a pain reliever by stimulating the adrenal gland.

ENHANCING POSITIVE FEELINGS

Sex can enhance positive feelings toward oneself and others. In giving and receiving tenderness and pleasure, one's positive outlook toward life is strengthened. As John Baum, M.D., professor of medicine at the University of Rochester, New York and author of a study examining the connection between stress and juvenile rheumatoid arthritis, notes a positive outlook is absolutely crucial to overcoming the obstacles presented by arthritis. In other words, the successful patient never gives up.

PARTICULAR PROBLEMS OF
THE PERSON WITH ARTHRITIS

The person with arthritis may not desire sexual intercourse due to pain, fatigue, anemia, or lack of interest. Ann Hamilton, and Clifford Hawkins, M.D. ("Sex and Arthritis", **Reports on Rheumatic Diseases, 1959-1977,** ARTHRITIS AND RHEUMATISM COUNCIL FOR RESEARCH), believe the person with arthritis should be told that such feelings are not unique and may affect most people at some point in their lives.

However, sexual intercourse for the person with arthritis is still possible, even when some pain and limitation of movement exists. If necessary, positions and techniques geared to the needs of the partners ought to be discussed calmly and rationally in the presence of a physician or trained counsellor. Whatever methods are used, both partners should keep in mind that kindness and sympathetic understanding are an important part of sex. When kindness and understanding are present, an acceptable adjustment to whatever difficulties are presented by the arthritis can certainly be achieved.

More detailed and graphic information is found in the pamphlet SEX CAN HELP ARTHRITIS, available upon request from The Institute for Research of Rheumatic Diseases, P.O. Box 955, New York, New York 10023. Please enclose $0.35 to cover costs.

Chapter XVI
DMSO
And Arthritis

*A*ccording to Patrick McGrady Sr., late science editor of the MEDICAL TRIBUNE, the grossly excessive amount of time and money required to make a drug marketable is causing the steep decline of American prestige in world-wide pharmacology.

DMSO, or dimethyl sulfoxide, is a prime example of a drug that has suffered unjust FDA harassment and persecution. Persecution persists in spite of the fact that many respected researchers have found DMSO safe and startlingly effective for the treatment of a wide range of diseases and ailments.

In the early 1960's, DMSO began to achieve an almost mythic underground status as a jack-of-all-trades-type drug. This substance, both plentiful and inexpensive, was described as an analgesic (pain-reliever), tranquillizer, collagen solvent, vasodilating agent (substance which widens blood vessels), anti-inflammatory agent and bacteriostatic (agent which retards bacterial growth).

In addition to being used in industry in the manufacture of paints, dyes, synthetic fibers and paint thinners, DMSO was also found to be an excellent anti-freeze and organ preservative.

Stanley W. Jacob, M.D., associate professor of surgery at the University of Oregon School of Medicine, was first introduced to DMSO by a colleague who heard about his search for a storage coolant for transplantable organs.

According to Pat McGrady, Dr. Jacob "fell in love with DMSO at first sight, smell and taste." After extensive animal testing, Dr. Jacob became convinced of the safety of DMSO, observing that topical, oral, rectal, intravenous and intraperitoneal administration were all safe and problem-free.

The Oregon-based surgeon and scientist later found DMSO extremely useful in the treatment of burns, severe bruises, swollen sprained ankles, "black eyes", frostbitten feet and hands, and sports-related trauma. Laboratory studies by other researchers demonstrated DMSO efficacy in selectively destroying leukemia cells, preventing and treating radiation injury, mildly dissolving enzymes and steroids, and obstructing the disease-causing activity of diverse microbes.

Significant improvement after DMSO administration was shown in two-thirds of a patient population with various forms of arthritis.

However, medical journals proved extremely reluctant to accept Dr. Jacob's assertions that DMSO was versatile in the treatment of burns, bursitis, and other ailments. Colleagues gave vent to hostility with ridicule.

On September 9, 1965, the WALL STREET JOURNAL published an article suggesting that DMSO may have caused the death of a 44-year old woman who had been taking the drug in an acceptable dosage along with penicillin and other substances. About seven weeks later — on November 10, 1965 — the FDA decided to halt all further research on DMSO. The World Health Organization and American embassies throughout the world were notified of this grave decision.

Despite the damage done by the WALL STREET JOURNAL article and subsequent harassment of Dr. Jacob by FDA officials, the New York Academy of Sciences agreed to sponsor an international symposium on DMSO on March 14, 15 and 16, 1966. Over a thousand researchers came from the United States and abroad to deliver papers dealing with this highly controversial substance.

Listed below are some of the key points made during the symposium.

1) Microorganisms found in CANCER and LEUKEMIA patients stopped growing when exposed to 25% DMSO (F. Seibert, Mound Park Hospital Foundation, St. Petersburg, Florida).

2) Depending on concentration, DMSO appeared to

control the dangers of clotting and bleeding (Herbert L. Davis, University of Nebraska College of Medicine).

3) When DMSO was added to cortisol and testosterone preparations, it enhanced skin penetration of these HORMONES 350% (Howard I. Maibach, University of California Medical Center, San Francisco).

4) Alone and combined with antibiotics like tetracycline DMSO produced good to excellent results in acute otitis media (inflammation of the middle ear), inflamed pus pockets in ear and nose, impetiginous eczema (skin ailment), pharyngitis, tonsilitis, aphthous stomatitis (inflammation of the mucous membrane of the mouth associated with small white spots), temporomandibular neuralgia (nerve pain in the region of the jaw's temporomandibular joint), hematoma (accumulation of blood under the skin), cold sores and shingles (Hans Asen, Berlin, Germany).

5) After open chest surgery, experimental subjects treated with DMSO had fewer complications, coughed more easily, had greater mobility in and out of bed, and required less morphine than control subjects. (Dale S. Penrod, Pennsylvania Hospital, Philadelphia).

6) When 187 patients with tendinitis, bursitis, strains and sprains, in an uncontrolled experiment and 92 others in a double-blind controlled experiment were treated with 60-90% DMSO or 10% DMSO as placebo, approximately 85 percent of the DMSO-treated patients showed good to excellent scores in improvement of pain, tenderness, edema, increase of movement, and of low side-effects, compared to none in the placebo group. (J.H. Brown, Seatt).

7) In a group of 500 patients with arthritic conditions, 70% responded well to topical administration of DMSO. Acute disorders cleared up totally. However, chronic conditions tended to respond favorably only during the course of treatment and for varying periods after treatment was terminated. Favorable responses were achieved with acute musculoskeletal disorders (81.1%), osetoarthritis (84.1% — during treatment!), rheumatoid arthritis (77.7%), acute tendinitis (94%), acute neuritis (88.2%), and acute synovitis (88%). The following parameters were evaluated: increased movement, reduced swelling, pain relief.

(Arthur Steinberg, Albert Einstein Medical Center).

8) Dr. Lester Persky, of University Hospitals, Cleveland, Ohio, and Dr. Stewart of the Cleveland Clinic, reported that two out of fifteen patients with interstitial cystitis, six out of thirteen with Peyronie's disease, disease of unknown origin which produces deformity and pain upon penile erection, two out of five patients with herpes progenitalis, two out of two with polycystic kidney pain, and one out of fourteen with vague genital pain all experienced improvement from DMSO therapy.

It took twelve years, until 1978, for the FDA to approve DMSO for use in the treatment of interstitial cystitis. The excessive restrictions placed on DMSO research in the area of interstitial cystitis were, ironically enough, based on studies in dogs, rabbits and swine given eye injections. Apparently, DMSO had been responsible for changes in the retinas of these experimental animals. However, comparable eye changes have not been observed in clinical studies involving human subjects. Prompted by FDA bureaucrats, the news media alleged that DMSO could cause blindness.

What is especially ironic about FDA approval of DMSO for use in interstitial cystitis therapy, is that this drug is equally or more effective in treating many other conditions. Between 1966 and 1978, DMSO remained in official limbo, although dedicated scientists continued to test the solvent's therapeutic efficacy upon the dread diseases of our time such as cardiovascular disease and stroke. Several medical centers participated in an animal study in which myocardial (heart muscle) scarring from myocardial fibrosis was reduced following DMSO treatment. Myocardial fibrosis is the formation of fibrous tissue, either as a reactive or healing process, in heart muscle tissue. Among the centers participating were the University of San Diego School of Medicine's department of pathology and the Hoffman-La Roche department of clinical pharmacology.

According to the researchers, whose results were published in the AMERICAN JOURNAL OF MEDICAL SCIENCE, the study suggests that DMSO can be useful in treating certain forms of myocardial injury and may even be of benefit in stiumlating the healing of myocardial infarcts resulting from coronary occlusion.

129

Dr. George E. Moore, acting head of surgery at Denver General Hospital, has used DMSO along with several other anti-cancer preparations to treat "accessible cancers". A veteran in the field of cancer treatment and tumor immunology, Dr. Moore feels that a significant mechanism of action of the DMSO-anti-cancer preparations was their ability to enhance immunity.

Jack C. de la Torre, Sc.D. of the University of Chicago School of Medicine, performed important work in decreasing the mortality and morbidity associated with spinal cord injury, stroke and brain trauma. Dr. de la Torre attempted to treat these conditions before damage became irreversible. DMSO was found to be effective in stimulating recovery and return to normal function.

At present, legislation in ten states permits a range of DMSO use. According to MEDICAL WORLD NEWS (October 11, 1982), Oregon, Florida and Louisiana are most liberal in the number of permissible applications.

FINAL WORDS: PROS AND CONS

At the New York Academy of Science's third conference on DMSO applications and actions, five American clinical reports, one from the Netherlands and one from Japan, suggest possible DMSO effectiveness in the treatment of amyloidosis. In amyloidosis, accumulation of amyloidosis a fine fibrillar protein takes place outside the cells of various organs and tissues of the body.

The September 1982 symposium produced both good and bad news. Ophthalmologist Charles A. Garcia of the University of Texas indicated no significant improvement in retinitis pigmentosa with DMSO treatment. In retinitis pigmentosa, a chronic and progressive inflammation of the retina is accompanied by atrophy and pigmentary infiltration of the inner layers of the eye. However, he also indicated no evidence of "ocular toxicity" from long-term use of DMSO at low dosages.

Frederick T. Waller, a neurosurgeon at Oregon Health Sciences University, reported that DMSO infusions raised intracranial pressure among 11 patients who did not respond favorably to conventional approaches such as, hyperventilation, fluid restriction, intravenous steriods and intravenous pentobarbital.

Dr. William M. Bennett administered DMSO as experimental therapy for stable spinal cord injuries and observed no kidney injury or decrease in renal function as a result of such therapy.

Finally, Dr. John B. Gelderd, associate professor of anatomy at Texas A & M University in College Station, reported that DMSO combined with hyperbaric oxygen, when started within 15 minutes of injury, appeared to be a viable "biological environment" for regeneration of nerve fibers after spinal cord injury.

Clearly, the final word on DMSO is not yet in. However, the amazing advances in DMSO research achieved despite FDA harassment and establishment shortsightedness prove once again that the dedication of researchers willing to take risks is never in vain.

Chapter XVII
The Case Against Immunization

*T*here has never been definitive proof that artificial immunization — the introduction of foreign proteins or live viruses into the bloodstream of whole populations — is either safe or effective.

Nor is it by any means clear that the many diseases for which new vaccines continue to be developed are threatening enough to justify compulsory mass inoculation.

Richard Moskowitz M.D. (JOURNAL OF THE NATIONAL CENTER FOR HOMEOPATHY, May and June, 1983) believes we have been taught to accept vaccination blindly without considering its long-term consequences for human health.

Flu, measles, mumps and poliomyelitis vaccines introduce viruses into the body and can trigger a wide range of diseases, including rheumatoid arthritis, lupus erythematosus, multiple sclerosis, Parkinson's disease and cancer, Dr. Robert Simpson of Rutgers University notes.

HOW EFFECTIVE ARE THE VARIOUS VACCINES?

Eminent medical authorities continue to question whether the marked decline in the prevalence and seriousness of many diseases can be attributed to the vaccines developed against them.

According to the epidemiologist C.C. Dauer (cited in HOSPITAL PRACTICE, October, 1980), whooping cough had already begun to decline long before the whooping cough (pertussis) vaccine became available.

Diphtheria and tetanus, as well as tuberculosis, cholera and typhoid also began to disappear at the end of the nineteenth century, probably as a response to sanitation and public health improvements.

NOT A REAL IMMUNITY

The main evidence that vaccines are effective dates from a period close to the present. During this time, the polio epidemics of the 1940's and 1950's were eliminated from developed nations. Following introduction of the MMR (mumps, measles, rubella) vaccine, these three diseases of childhood have become much less prevalent.

It is by no means certain that these vaccines produce an authentic continuous immunity, however, since the diseases against which they were devised have continued to erupt in highly immunized populations.

PERTUSSIS (WHOOPING COUGH) VACCINE

According to G. Stewart ("Vaccination Against Whooping Cough; Efficiency vs. Risks", LANCET, 1977), in a recent British outbreak of whooping cough **completely immunized children** developed the disease in large numbers. Also, according to Dr. Stewart (NEW ENGLAND JOURNAL OF MEDICINE), 30-50% of recent cases of pertussis — including some studied at the United States Center for Disease Control in Atlanta, Georgia — occurred in children WHO HAD ALREADY RECEIVED THREE OR MORE INJECTIONS OF VACCINE!

Pertussis vaccine may cause serious fevers, convulsions and brain injury (encephalopathy). Because of these dangers, most public health officials forbid its use after age six.

MEASLES VACCINE

In 1977, thirty-four cases of measles were observed at the University of California at Los Angeles in a college population that was deemed 91% immune!

Measles vaccine is supposed to prevent the development

of measles encephalitis, which occurs in about 1 out of every 10,000 or 100,000 cases of measles.

However, measles vaccine is known to cause brain damage in one case out of every million and has been linked to such serious and sometimes fatal conditions as aseptic meningitis, seizure disorders, retardation, paralysis of one side of the body, learning disorders, hyperactivity and ataxia, inability to coordinate muscle movements.

Hillas Smith, M.D. ("Measles Again," THE LANCET) holds the view that perhaps only extremely weakened children should be immunized against measles, considering the risks connected with immunization. These children might include those with chronic respiratory disease, Down's syndrome, or severe malnutrition.

The unnecessary high costs of routine vaccination and blood testing could be sharply reduced.

German measles (rubella) vaccine is of extremely doubtful value and may produce arthritis.

SMALLPOX VACCINE

Smallpox immunization has finally been abandoned because life-threatening dangers from the vaccine were found to be higher than risks from smallpox itself.

These dangers include encephalitis, inflammation of the brain, eczema vaccinatum, an inflammatory condition of the skin characterized by blisters on the face and neck, high fever, and enlargement of the lymph nodes, and progressive vaccinia' which can cause death. The death rate of all these conditions is high.

DIPHTHERIA VACCINE

Though once fatal, diphtheria has been almost completely eliminated but immunization continues.

According to Robert S. Mendelsohn M.D. (THE PEOPLE'S DOCTOR Newsletter, "The Truth About Immunization," Volume 2, Number 4), diphtheria immunization is of doubtful value even when diphtheria does occur. In a 1969 outbreak of the disease in Chicago, a Chicago Board of Health

Report indicated that four of the sixteen victims had been thoroughly immunized and five others had received at least one dose of the vaccine!

POLIOMYELITIS VACCINE

In 1977 Jonas Salk, M.D., developer of the killed polio virus vaccine, stated that since the early 1970's, the majority of cases of polio in the United States were probably caused by live polio vaccine which is no longer in use.

INFLUENZA VACCINE

According to Dr. Albert Sabin, co-developer of the oral polio vaccine and Distinguished Professor of Biomedicine at the Medical University of South Carolina in Charleston, there is no **justification** for giving influenza vaccine to any age group.

Most "flu" is in fact caused by viruses distinct from varieties of the influenza-A virus. There is strong evidence that the elderly receive scant protection from the vaccine, which should only be used for authentic epidemics.

In 1976, 565 cases of Guillain-Barre paralysis were traced to swine flu vaccine. In addition, there were thirty mysterious deaths from swine flu vaccine.

"BOOSTER" SHOTS

On the basis of some of the above data, one might assume that vaccines confer only temporary immunity which must be buttressed at regular intervals by "booster" shots. This notion, however, is questionable from several perspectives.

A number of researchers have shown (J. Cherry, "The New Epidemiology of Measles and Rubella," HOSPITAL PRACTICE, July 1980) that when a person inoculated against measles develops the disease, "boosters" are virtually without effect.

In addition, vaccines do not act simply by inducing mild copies of the disease in question. The illnesses they produce may be far more harmful than the original disease. In a recent outbreak of mumps among supposedly immune schoolchildren,

135

several **uncommon** symptoms, including vomiting, rashes and anorexia, or aversion to food, developed.

Vaccines have also been known to produce cases of measles involving complications of pneumonia, arthritis, pinpoint hemorrhages (petechiae), swelling and severe pain which were far more serious than the typical form of the disease.

A PHYSICIAN'S PERSONAL EXPERIENCE WITH VACCINE-RELATED ILLNESS

Dr. Moskowitz has had extensive experience with disease caused by vaccines. He has encountered at least half a dozen cases of children who developed several symptoms — fevers, irritability, temper tantrums, as well as enhanced susceptibility to colds, ear infections and tonsillitis — which were traced to pertussis vaccine.

One five-year-old boy developed leukemia following his first pertussis (DPT) vaccination. According to the boy's family doctor, he had been successfully treated with natural remedies on two previous occasions but complete relapse occurred after each successive DPT booster. As if this connection between leukemia and routine vaccination is not scandalous enough, the physician admitted that he had not dared to admit his suspicions concerning vaccine-related leukemia to the boy's parents.

Due to a similar lack of courage on the part of medical practitioners regarding the dangers of vaccination, the general public is being deprived of crucial information.

Dr. Moskowitz also observed blood changes suggestive of leukemia in a 9½-month-old girl who had received the whooping cough vaccine. There were no cough or clearcut respiratory symptoms. This suggests that when introduced directly into the blood, the whooping cough vaccine may stimulate disease on a more systemic level rather than allowing the whooping cough bacterium to produce inflammatory symptoms only in the nose or mouth area.

Leukemia is a cancerous invasion of the blood and blood-forming organs — liver, spleen, lymph nodes and bone marrow. These organs are also the basic components of the body's immune system. If vaccines do indeed work **against** the body on a systemic level, it is logical that they would attack the immune system.

DEVELOPING A THEORY ON
THE BASIS OF THE DATA

As a result of his extensive experience with vaccine-related disease, Dr. Moskowitz believes that vaccination may in fact drive the disease deeper into our bodies instead of protecting us against disease. As a result of harboring the disease chronically, our responses become weaker and weaker. The disease then shows a reduced tendency to heal.

THE NATURAL RESPONSE TO DISEASE

Let us first consider a natural response to measles, mainly a disease of the respiratory tract. Infected droplets in the air are produced by the sneezing and coughing of a person with measles.

The measles virus multiplies in the tonsils, adenoids and lymph tissues of the naso-pharynx of the susceptible person who inhales these droplets. Multiplication continues in the lymph nodes of the neck and head, and ends in the thymus and bone marrow, key organs of the immune system. During the ten-to-fourteen day incubation period, the patient experiences few symptoms.

At the time the first symptoms appear, antibodies can be found in the blood. Antibodies produced by the immune system are the body's first line of defense against foreign invaders such as bacteria and viruses. When the number of circulating antibodies is at its height, the intensity of symptoms is also greatest. This means that the measles "illness" is merely the immune system's major effort to rid the blood of the measles virus.

When the disease is allowed to follow its natural course, the virus is removed by the same routes through which is entered — sneezing and coughing.

Under normal circumstances, developing and recovering from a disease like measles involves the recruitment of the whole immune system, e.g. inflammation and activation of white blood cells and scavenger cells called macrophages. Antibody production is just one facet of the whole process.

137

As indicated by C. Phillips ("Measles", in V. Vaughan, NELSON'S TEXTBOOK OF PEDIATRICS, Saunders, 1979), a child who recovers from measles **naturally** will never be susceptible to it again. Having combated the disease successfully, he or she will also succeed in responding effectively to all future infections.

THE ARTIFICIAL (VACCINE) APPROACH
TO FIGHTING DISEASE

In contrast, when an artificially-attenuated (weakened) virus is injected into the blood directly, it does not trigger a general inflammation or any of the other defense mechanisms that enable us to respond vigorously and soundly to infection.

Instead, the weakened virus gains immediate access to the major immune tissues leaving no obvious route to expel the virus. The virus may remain in the blood permanently causing a progressive weakening of the capacity to respond adequately not only to this particular virus but to all infections.

Rather than producing authentic immunity, vaccines or artificial immunization, obstruct and suppress the immune system just as chemotherapy and radiation do. Antibodies are produced but antibody production is just one aspect of the immune response to disease and cannot stand in for the entire immune process.

Under these circumstances, the virus survives as a foreign element within the cells of the immune system and creates a chronic disease. The virus becomes completely attached to the host cell's genetic material. Then the immune system tries to produce antibodies against these viruses, it ends up directing these antibodies against its own cells and destroying them.

This condition, in which it becomes impossible for the body to recognize its own cells or get rid of foreign invaders like viruses, is called chronic immune failure or chronic immune deficiency.

TUMOR FORMATION:
ADVANCED STAGE OF CHRONIC IMMUNE FAILURE

Tumor formation — cancer — might be considered an advanced stage of chronic immune failure in which cells chronically infected by viruses and other invaders begin to multiply independently.

YOUR RIGHT TO REFUSE
IMMUNIZATION IN FOREIGN TRAVEL

No one must undergo immunization or vaccination when travelling abroad.

Some uninformed public health officials continue to claim, however, that it is impossible to travel outside the United States without certain immunizations.

As pointed out by Clinton R. Miller, National Health Federation representative (THE NATIONAL HEALTH FEDERATION BULLETIN, Volume X, Number 12), thousands of unimmunized travellers pass in and out of the United States each year without difficulty or inconvenience. With improvement in health standards in other countries all over the world, there is less and less need for immunization.

If you do plan to travel out of the country, awareness of your rights can help in dealing with misinformed public health officials.

Along with a passport application, an immunization certificate is also given to the person planning to travel.

The immunization certificate must be completed by your immunizing physician and stamped with the stamp of the local or state health officer situated in the area of the immunizing physician only if you have been immunized.

You do not have to show vaccination for any disease on the form in order to leave or re-enter the United States.

ADVICE FROM HEALTH OFFICIALS

When departing, if you ask for information from a public health official, you may be encouraged to undergo vaccination — WITHOUT BEING TOLD, HOWEVER, ABOUT THE SERIOUS SIDE EFFECTS AND RISKS OF IMMUNIZATION! The immunization official may even inform you that vaccination will make re-entry into the United States much easier.

If this is the case, state politely but firmly that you intend to depart from and return to the United States **unvaccinated.** You are very much within your rights.

Although vaccination will be offered on your return, you are under no obligation to accept. Even if you have just left a country afflicted with smallpox epidemic, you are not required to undergo vaccination.

However, the medical officer, in appraising the risk he or she thinks you represent, may decide to put you under surveillance. Under these circumstances, you return unvaccinated to your home town. You are then required to report regularly for a period of up to fourteen days from the time of departure from the foreign country to your local health official so that suspicious symptoms do not go undetected and untreated. If you observe any outbreaks on your own, you must report for quarantine or isolation.

Note: If there have been outbreaks of smallpox aboard ship or in the last foreign country visited, the vaccinated person may be asked to submit to the same surveillance procedures as the unvaccinated person. The vaccinated person, then, is by no means exempt.

Quarantine, or isolation, is very very rarely used. It simply means that you are isolated in a house for no more then two weeks with room and board paid for by the government. As with surveillance, the vaccinated person is no more exempt from the possibility of isolation than the unvaccinated person.